UNRAVELING THE SELF:
A PATH TO PERSONAL GROWTH

BY
ASTRID AUXIER

© MEKIKI MAGAZINE

First published in English in 2023 By Mekiki Magazine
Copyright for the first English edition © 2023 Mekiki Magazine
Site: www.mekikimagazine.com

All rights reserved. No part of this publication may be reproduced, stored in a retrieval system, or transmitted in any form or by any means, electronic, mechanical, photocopying, recording, or otherwise, without the prior consent of the publisher. The author has made every effort to provide accurate information at the time of publication; neither the publisher nor the author assumes any responsibility for errors or for changes that occur after publication. Further, the publisher does not have any control over and does not assume any responsibility for the author or third-party websites or their content.

ISBN: 978-1-954145-55-9

Title: Unraveling The Self: A Path To Personal Growth
Author: Astrid Auxier
Editors: Mekiki and A. Lee

Book Cover By: Álvaro Oliveira For Mekiki Magazine
Graphic Design: Álvaro Oliveira For Mekiki Magazine

As the author, I want to disclose that I employ AI tools to aid in the editing and improvement of my writing. These AI tools, including editing, grammar, and spell-checking, assist me in enhancing the quality and readability of my work. However, it is essential to acknowledge that automated systems are not infallible. While I strive for accuracy and clarity in my writing, it is advisable for readers to exercise their own judgment and critical thinking. My commitment remains focused on providing the best possible reading experience, and I sincerely appreciate your understanding and support in this endeavor.

contents:

08 INTRODUCTION

12 CHAPTER I
Mindfulness, Acceptance, and Personal Growth as a Triad to Shape Our Lives

16 CHAPTER II
The Burdens of the Past and the Uncertainties of the Future

20 CHAPTER III
The Toll of Rumination and Anxiety

24 CHAPTER IV
Confronting the Past and Embracing the Future

28 CHAPTER V
The Power of the Present Moment

32 CHAPTER VI
Seizing the Potential of the Now

36	**CHAPTER VII** The Art of Mastering Our Actions, Choices, and Perspectives
39	**CHAPTER VIII** Mastering Mindfulness with Grace and Intention
42	**CHAPTER IX** Mindfulness Techniques to Stay Grounded and Focused
53	**CHAPTER X** The Long-Term Benefits of Mindfulness
65	**CHAPTER XI** A Cautionary Tale of Hubris and Ignorance
69	**CHAPTER XII** Deconstructing the Breathtaking Assumption of Linear Time
73	**CHAPTER XIII** Confronting Our Dislike for Unforeseen Outcomes

77	**CHAPTER XIV** Leveraging Acceptance to Reconcile the Past and the Present
80	**CHAPTER XV** The Alchemy of Acceptance and Unburdening the Soul
92	**CHAPTER XVI** The Elixir and Rewards of Acceptance
102	**CHAPTER XVII** The Eternal Present and Embracing the Moment
112	**CHAPTER XVIII** Navigating the Currents of Time With Mindful Anchors
125	**CHAPTER XIX** Balancing Acceptance and Change With the Scales of Serenity
136	**CHAPTER XX** Nurturing Empathy and Compassion on the Path to Growth and Connection
149	**CHAPTER XXI** Practical Empathic Strategies for Cultivating Emotional Intelligence
166	**CHAPTER XXII** Setting Realistic Goals for Personal Growth and Self-Improvement

186	**CHAPTER XXIII**	Practical Steps for Turning Long-Term Goals Into Manageable Tasks
205	**CHAPTER XXIV**	Embracing Change in the Face of Life's Uncertainties
223	**CHAPTER XXV**	Building Steadfast Resilience and Nurturing Personal Growth
243	**CHAPTER XXVI**	Practical Strategies for Reigniting Inner Evolution
260	**CHAPTER XXVII**	The Eternal Learning of the Mirrored Soul
271	**EPILOGUE**	
276	**OUR VISION**	
280	**AUTHOR'S BIOGRAPHY**	

Introduction

Perhaps you, too, have noticed that as the myriad threads of time weave an intricate tapestry of existence, it is easy to become entangled in the labyrinthine complexities that define our lives.

Inescapably, the relentless current of time carries with it the burdens of the past, the uncertainties of the future, and the delicate interplay of emotions that lay at the very core of the human experience. Yet, within this ever-shifting landscape, we can ultimately learn to navigate the treacherous waters of regret and worry and, in doing so, chart an exciting course toward a more fulfilling and meaningful existence.

With that in mind, in this humble tome, I shall endeavor to illuminate how anyone might claim a deeper understanding of a reverence for and a familiarity with the present moment and its profound impact on our lives. I will attempt to build a complex and layered melody that, through gentle choruses of reinforcement, provides all you need to thrive and prosper.

By peering through the unifying lens of mindfulness and acceptance, together, we will unravel the intricate threads that bind us to the past and the future, revealing the transformative power that lies dormant within the eternal present, simply waiting to be harnessed.

Peeling back further layers and exploring the multifaceted nature of the human condition, we shall delve into the delicate balance between arrogance and humility, acceptance and change, and, vitally, the inescapable passage of time. By examining the various manifestations of these emotions and their consequences, I aim to provide you, my most welcome reader, with the tools necessary to forge a new path forward, guided by the light of self-awareness and comfort in personal growth.

As we embark upon this journey, I fervently hope that the insights gleaned from these pages will serve as a beacon, guiding your journey toward understanding the present moment and its profound implications. Better yet, I seek not only to unlock the mysteries of self-improvement and emotional well-being but also to foster a sense of compassion and empathy that may yet ripple outwards, touching the lives of others.

And so, dear reader, I invite you to join me on this voyage through the shifting sands of human emotion. As we traverse this uncharted terrain, may we find solace, knowing that it is within our grasp to shape the course of our lives and the world around us. Only by embracing the present moment can we genuinely begin to untangle the intricate threads that bind us and, in doing so, weave a new tapestry of existence marked by wisdom, awareness, and the indomitable spirit of the human heart.

I.
Mindfulness, Acceptance, and Personal Growth as a Triad to Shape Our Lives

In the grand symphony of life, it is the interplay of seemingly disparate elements that coalesce to create a harmonious whole. Among these elements, mindfulness, acceptance, and personal growth emerge a powerful triad of distinct yet interconnected forces. As we navigate the tumultuous tides of existence, the delicate balance shared among these three forces holds the key to unlocking our full potential and ultimately seizing the ability to steer life on our own terms.

The first movement in this symphony is mindfulness or the art of cultivating a heightened awareness of the present moment. With its roots in ancient philosophy, mindfulness has emerged as an interesting tool for the modern era, offering solace and clarity amidst the relentless cacophony of our fast-paced world.

By embracing mindfulness, we can learn to attune ourselves to the subtle melodies of life and, in doing so, develop a profound sense of connection with ourselves, others, and the world we move through.

Yet mindfulness alone, while a potent force, is inadequate to weave a self-determined life tapestry. Instead, it requires the accompaniment of acceptance, the second movement in this symphony, through which we can learn to embrace the imperfections and uncertainties that define our innate humanity. As we confront the swirling maelstrom of our emotions, thoughts, and experiences, acceptance offers us a haven, a place where we can find solace and understanding amidst the storm.

With two strong footholds manifested in our quest to form a firm foundation, we have strength but not yet stability. That is because acceptance is not an end in itself but rather a stepping stone on the path toward the third and final movement of this symphony: personal growth.

As we master the transformative power of mindfulness and acceptance combined, we can begin to unlock the boundless potential for growth that lies within each of us, foundationally setting the stage for profound change and self-improvement.

The symbiotic balance between this trio of forces is a complex and ever-evolving dance, a dynamic interplay that shapes the course of our lives. As we embrace mindfulness, acceptance, and personal growth, we must also recognize the interwoven nature of these elements and the importance of nurturing each for the betterment of the whole.

> **By cultivating mindfulness, we can develop the self-awareness necessary to identify the areas in our lives that require attention and change. Through acceptance, we can learn to embrace these imperfections and the inherent uncertainty of life, finding solace and understanding amidst the chaos. And finally, by tending to our personal growth, we can transcend prior obstacles to realize a more freely flowing form of self-improvement fueled by everything we have gleaned from our journey thus far.**

II.
The Burdens of the Past and the Uncertainties of the Future

As the hands of time march inexorably forward, we find ourselves inextricably entwined with the past and the future. The complexities of our existence are bound to these temporal realms, shaped by our memories and aspirations.

It is in this elaborate tangle of past and future that we often find ourselves ensnared as we dwell on bygone days and fret over the unknowables that lie ahead. It is a common human tendency that often leaves us shackled to the weight of history and gripped with fear for what may come, one that is, however, graciously annullable when we climb successfully to a more advantageous vantage point.

In our quest to navigate the interlacing passageways of time, we often become mired in the past's quagmire. The echoes of our memories reverberate in the caverns of our minds, shaping our identities and coloring our perceptions of the world around us.

While the past can serve as a fertile ground for growth and self-discovery, it can also trap us in a web of regret and longing. The specters of missed opportunities haunt us, past mistakes and relationships that have slid from our trajectory. As we grapple with the burdens of the past, the uncertainties of the future loom large on the horizon.

This reminds us that the future, an ever-shifting patchwork of possibilities, is a fickle and capricious mistress, forever eluding our grasp. We yearn for the comfort of certainty, of knowing what fate has in store for us. Yet, in our pursuit of this elusive quarry, anxiety and fear often beset us as we attempt to peer through the veil that obscures our destiny.

It is precisely this dual struggle with the past and the future that forms the backdrop of the human experience, a waltz of longing and fear that spans the ages. Yet, it is precisely within this lowland that we find the seeds of transformation, the potential for growth and self-discovery that await its opportunity to sprout.

As we learn to navigate smoothly through and past these burdens, we can begin to loosen the bonds that tether us to the past and the future and, in doing so, chart a course toward higher ground and the reward of a more fulfilling and meaningful existence.

> **In the chapters that follow, we shall embark upon a journey through the mists of time, exploring the human psyche and its relationship to the temporal realms. By plunging into the depths of our memories and confronting the unquantifiable future, we will collect the tools and wisdom necessary to move knowingly toward our highest selves.**

III.
The Toll of Rumination and Anxiety

Before mastering how to shed life's burdens, there is immense value in understanding why the need to carry such weights is an illusion. We must recognize that as we progress through life, the lingering stories of the past and the uncertainties of the future often cast long shadows over our minds, weaving rumination and anxiety into our personal tapestries.

These twin specters, though seemingly distinct from one another, are our collaborative opponents and their insidious grip on our thoughts and emotions can exact a heavy toll on our personal well-being and relationships.

Speaking of duality, rumination, the act of dwelling on past events or emotions, can be a double-edged sword. While reflection and introspection can offer valuable insights and foster growth, excessive rumination can lead to a downward spiral of negative thoughts and emotions. This unrelenting focus on the past can erode our sense of self-worth, fuel feelings of regret and guilt, and ultimately impair our ability to function and thrive in the present.

Anxiety, the uneasy companion of rumination, is a pervasive force that often stems from our preoccupation with the uncontrollable future. Fearful of what may come, we find ourselves trapped in a cycle of worry and apprehension, our minds consumed by countless "what if" scenarios.

This constant state of disquiet can have unwelcome consequences for our mental and emotional well-being, manifesting in a myriad of ways, including chronic stress, sleep disturbances, and even physical ailments.

As we grapple with the weight of rumination and anxiety, our relationships with others are not immune to their effects. The persistent cloud of negativity and worry that accompanies these mental states can create an emotional barrier, distancing us from the very people we hold dear. Our capacity for empathy, understanding, and genuine connection can become compromised as we struggle to maintain our emotional equilibrium amidst the turbulence of our own thoughts and feelings.

Yet, it is only in knowing and seeing both rumination and anxiety that we can begin the work of peeling them away. By recognizing the impact of these mental states on our well-being and relationships, we can start to develop the tools and strategies necessary to loosen their grip. Upon our sturdy foundation of mindfulness, acceptance, and personal growth, we can break patterns of thought and behavior that have been preventing our ascension.

IV.
Confronting the Past and Embracing the Future

As we begin to see the patterns that uniquely shape our experiential tapestries, it becomes increasingly apparent that achieving a balance between acknowledging the past and embracing the future is of paramount importance. The past, with its myriad lessons and experiences, and the future, with its boundless potential and possibility, can play a critical role both in hindering or enhancing our personal growth and well-being.

To fully confront the past, we must first recognize the influence it holds over our lives. Then, through self-reflection and introspection, we can begin to unravel the tangled strands of our memories, gaining valuable insights and understanding from the experiences that have shaped us.

By illuminating and acknowledging the lessons and wisdom gleaned from our past, we can cultivate a sense of gratitude for the journey we have undertaken while also fostering the resilience necessary to overcome the challenges that lie ahead.

However, confronting the past must not become an exercise in rumination or self-flagellation. It is crucial to strike a balance between learning from our experiences and becoming mired in the marshlands of regret and guilt. By practicing self-compassion and forgiveness, we can learn to accept our past as an integral part of our story, which has molded us into the individuals we are today.

Simultaneously, embracing the uncertainties of the future is a vital aspect of our emotional well-being. The future, with its infinite potential, can be both exhilarating and terrifying in equal measure. By cultivating a sense of curiosity and wonder for the unknown, we can transform the anxiety and fear that often accompany thoughts of the future's ambiguities into a source of inspiration and growth.

To achieve this, we must learn to recognize that the future is a vast and unpredictable landscape that cannot be fully controlled or anticipated and develop a healthy relationship with the unknown. By cultivating a sense of adaptability and flexibility, we can learn to navigate future terrain as it forms with grace and resilience, viewing each unexpected twist and turn as an opportunity for self-discovery.

V.

The Power of the Present Moment

As the sun languidly begins its descent towards the horizon, painting the sky with hues of crimson and gold, it is impossible not to be struck by the transient beauty of the moment. This ephemeral quality, the fleeting nature of each instant as it slips through our fingers like grains of sand, serves as a poignant reminder of the inescapable passage of time, for it is time's perpetual current that sweeps us forward, also carrying the burdens of our past and the uncertainties of our future along if we fail to release them from the nets that hang in our wake.

In this inexorable propulsion, one finds that a pervasive preoccupation with the shadowy recesses of the past and the hazy vistas of the future often defines the human condition. Consumed by these distant visions, we frequently overlook the one realm in which we can genuinely make an extraordinary impact—the eternal now.

The present moment, so often neglected, holds within its embrace the power to reshape our lives with staggering vigor and dynamism. It is here, at the heart of the ever-changing tableau of existence, that we can take control of our destinies and begin the meaningful work of self-improvement and personal growth, for it is only in the present that we can gain confident control of our relationships with the specters of our past and uncertainties of our future, ultimately, freeing ourselves from the shackles of time.

Yet, to pluck this opportunity, we must first learn to navigate the labyrinthine corridors of the present and, in doing so, cultivate the skills necessary to harness its transformative power. The key to unlocking this potential lies in the art of mindfulness, the practice of maintaining a state of heightened awareness and self-reflection in the face of the ceaseless ebb and flow of life.

By embracing mindfulness, we can learn to anchor ourselves in the now, cultivating a sense of calm and focus that allows us to flow through the myriad challenges that we encounter each day. In this tranquil state, we can begin to untangle the complex web of emotions, thoughts, and actions that define our existence and, in doing so, discover new threads that we might choose to weave with greater intention, such as understanding, empathy, and resilience.

As our explorations take us further into the realm of the present, we must also learn to balance the delicate interplay between acceptance and change.

While it is true that the past is immutable and the future uncertain, the present offers us the opportunity to shape our reality through our actions, choices, and perspective. By cultivating a spirit of acceptance, we can learn to reconcile ourselves with the events of our past while also embracing the potential for change that lies readily within each moment.

> **And so, returning to the sun's departing crimson rays, let us pause to reflect upon the eternal present and the role it plays in shaping our lives. In essence, we cannot escape the onward motion of the now, but we can make our home within it as it shifts and swirls around us, seeing with eyes that are fully open to its untold opportunities for both rest and self-creation.**

VI.

Seizing the Potential of the Now

As we draw the power of the present moment into greater focus, we begin to uncover its substantial potential as a place from which personal growth and self-improvement can spring. It is in the realm of the now that we have the capacity to rewrite our stories, redefine our identities, and adjust our course toward self-actualization.

With its infinite possibilities, the present moment offers a direct line to growth and self-discovery. By developing a keen awareness of our thoughts, emotions, and experiences, we can identify the areas of our lives that require attention and nurturing.

This heightened state of self-awareness enables us to tap into our inner resources, unlocking the wisdom, resilience, and strength necessary to surmount the self-constructed barriers and challenges that stand in our way.

To harness the transformative power of the present moment, we must first commit to a process of introspection and self-assessment. This begins with a candid evaluation of our current circumstances, acknowledging both our strengths and areas in need of improvement.

By cultivating a sense of self-compassion and self-acceptance, we can approach this process with honesty and humility, recognizing that personal growth is an ongoing journey marked by both triumphs and setbacks.

Next, we must establish a clear vision for our desired future, setting realistic and attainable goals that align with our deepest values and aspirations. In doing so, we create a roadmap for our journey, providing a sense of direction and purpose as we navigate each day's unique twists and turns.

The metamorphic potential of the present moment is further amplified through the practice of mindfulness and intentional living. By cultivating a deep sense of presence and attentiveness, we can learn to recognize the opportunities for growth and self-improvement that may otherwise pass us by. Moreover, this mindful approach to living empowers us to make conscious choices and take deliberate action, fostering a sense of agency and mastery over our destinies, no matter the parameters that remain outside our control.

VII.
The Art of Mastering Our Actions, Choices, and Perspectives

In the grand and motley mosaic of life, it is often the seemingly inconsequential actions, choices, and perspectives that we adopt in the present moment that bears the most significant impact on the trajectory of our lives. Though often overlooked, the subtle decisions we make and the viewpoints we embrace possess a remarkable capacity to shape distant outcomes and mold the essence of our being.

That is precisely why it is within the domain of the present that we must seize the reins of our lives, taking control of our actions, choices, and perspectives with intentionality, wisdom, and courage.

Mastering our actions begins with strengthening and flexing our metaphorical muscles of self-awareness and self-discipline. By honing our ability to attune to our thoughts, emotions, and experiences, we can develop a keen understanding of the underlying motives, assumptions, and desires that drive our actions. Moreover, this heightened self-awareness enables us to make more informed decisions rooted in our core values and principles as we navigate each new experience.

With practice, we soon realize that each choice, whether large or small, holds the potential for growth, self-discovery, and strategic transformation within it. By exercising intentionality and discernment in our decision-making, we can trigger a cascade of positive change, both within ourselves and in the lives of those we touch.

Our perspectives also play a critical role in determining the course of our lives. The lens through which we view the world colors our perspective on events, influencing our thoughts, emotions, and actions in a myriad of ways.

> **By adopting a more flexible and adaptive mindset, we can see challenges and setbacks as opportunities for growth and learning rather than insurmountable obstacles. This shift in inner seeing can facilitate a liberating and empowering reframing, imbuing even the most difficult circumstances with meaning and purpose.**

VIII.
Mastering Mindfulness with Grace and Intention

One concept stands as a cornerstone in our pursuit of self-mastery and personal growth; an essential practice that offers a gateway to a more mindful, present, and intentional existence: the art of mindfulness. This ancient discipline, with its roots firmly planted in the wisdom of the ages, offers us a means to navigate the complexities of our lives with a heightened sense of presence, awareness, and grace.

At its core, mindfulness is the practice of paying deliberate and non-judgmental attention to the present moment. By focusing our awareness on our thoughts, emotions, sensations, and experiences as they unfold, we cultivate a deeper connection to the richness and beauty of the here and now. This heightened sense of presence enables us to engage more fully with our lives, fostering a greater sense of curiosity, wonder, and appreciation for the world.

The significance of mindfulness in embracing the present moment cannot be overstated. Through the practice of mindfulness, we are better equipped to steer the present rather than being pulled along by it, making it a space of sanctuary rather than turbulence.

By learning to quiet the cacophony of thoughts, emotions, and distractions that so often cloud our minds, we can uncover a wellspring of inner peace, resilience, and clarity, allowing us to approach our lives with that vital intentionality, alongside a softness of wisdom and grace.

> **Practicing mindfulness also reinforces our foundation for personal growth and self-improvement. By developing a deeper understanding of our thoughts, emotions, and behaviors through the simple practice of mindful self-observation, we can identify the patterns and habits that may be hindering our progress or causing us unnecessary suffering. Armed with this newfound awareness, we can take deliberate and focused action to change these patterns, fostering true agency over our own lives.**

IX.
Mindfulness Techniques to Stay Grounded and Focused

It is no small feat to remain grounded and focused in a world that constantly bathes us in a dissonance of distractions. Yet, with its diverse array of techniques and practices, the art of mindfulness clears a path toward tranquility and presence amidst the chaos of our modern lives. To help you harness this resource, in this chapter, we shall explore a curated selection of mindfulness techniques designed to help individuals remain centered, attentive, and fully engaged in the present moment.

❶ The Breath as an Anchor

Few among us are strangers to the whirlwind of thoughts and emotions that can descend upon one's mind, particularly in moments of high stress or uncertainty. We can find solace and grounding in the simple yet profound practice of conscious breathing.

Allow me to share a personal anecdote with you, dear reader, that illustrates the transformative power of this practice. I recall a particularly challenging period in my life, fraught with deadlines, creative blocks, and personal turmoil. I found myself caught in the maelstrom of my thoughts, unable to find a moment of peace from the noise.

One evening, as I sat at my writing desk, my mind racing and my heart heavy, I decided, on the example of the sages, to turn my attention to my breath. With each inhalation and exhalation, I felt the weight of my worries and fears gradually begin to dissipate, replaced by a newfound sense of stillness and tranquility.

As I continued to focus on the sensation of my breath entering and leaving my body, I discovered a haven of serenity within the storm, a grounding force that served as a constant reminder of the present moment. My breath became my anchor, a lifeline that guided me back to the shores of my own awareness time and time again.

This practice of conscious breathing, so deceptively simple in its execution, has since become an invaluable tool not only in my quest for inner peace and clarity but also in those of countless others. Through the cultivation of presence and stillness, we can learn to dispel anxiety and meet each moment with an open heart and a tranquil mind.

So I invite you to explore the transformative power of the breath as an anchor in your own life. In moments of chaos or uncertainty, allow yourself to be drawn back to the present moment through the simple act of conscious breathing.

You may find, as I have, that by directing your attention to the sensation of your breath as it flows in and out of your body, you discover a key that unlocks one of many doors to a greater sense of peace, presence, and stillness, even in the most tumultuous of circumstances.

❷ Body Scan Meditation

Life often demands a great deal of mental and emotional engagement, leaving us feeling disconnected from the very vessels that carry us through life. In my personal journey towards greater self-awareness and presence, I have discovered a practice that has profoundly impacted my ability to reconnect with my physical self: the body scan meditation.

Knowing this, I'd like to share with you a moment of revelation, one that illuminated the power of this seemingly unassuming technique.

It was during a retreat, far removed from the clamor of my everyday life that I first experienced the body scan meditation. As I lay on my back, eyes closed, the gentle voice of the meditation guide beckoned me to direct my attention to my feet, encouraging me to observe any sensations that arose without judgment or attachment.

As I continued to follow the guidance, slowly moving my focus up through my legs, my torso, and eventually to my head, I became acutely aware of the subtle sensations within my body. The tingling of my toes, the warmth of my breath on my upper lip, the gentle rise and fall of my chest—every part of my being seemed to come alive with a newfound sense of presence and vitality.

This intimate exploration of my physical self revealed not only a deeper connection to my body but also a profound sense of relaxation and calm. As I lay there, bathed in the experience's afterglow, I realized the immense value that lay within this simple practice. By grounding my awareness in the present moment and cultivating a non-judgmental curiosity toward my physical sensations, I unlocked yet another door to tranquility and connection.

Since that fateful day, the body scan meditation has become integral to my mindfulness practice. In moments of tension or disconnection, I return to this technique, allowing the often surprising and previously unnoticed interplay of sensations within my body to anchor me firmly in the present moment.

The practice of body scan meditation involves systematically directing our attention to different parts of the body while observing the sensations and experiences that arise in each area without judgment or attachment. This technique promotes a deep sense of relaxation and connection with our physical selves, grounding our awareness firmly in the present moment.

So why not explore the transformative potential of the body scan meditation in your own life? By fostering a deeper connection with your physical self and grounding your awareness in the present moment, you may find that this practice is a powerful antidote to the stresses and distractions that so often pull us away from the here and now.

❸ **Mindful Walking**

When our days are consumed by a ceaseless torrent of thoughts, words, and ideas, leaving little opportunity for a reprieve, we can claim an island of calm in the simple practice of mindful walking.

The first time I became aware of the potential of this technique, I had been wandering the verdant gardens of a secluded estate. As I indulged myself, meandering along a winding path, my gaze fell upon a single, dew-speckled leaf that lay suspended in the air, caught unusually in the breeze.

In that instant, I found myself fully and irrevocably present, my attention captivated by the simple beauty of the scene before me and my mind entirely absent of racing thoughts. With a deep inhalation, I resolved to maintain this newfound sense of presence as I continued my walk, focusing my attention on the subtle sensory medley that accompanied each step I took.

As I proceeded, I became acutely aware of the gentle caress of the wind against my skin, the rhythmic sound of my footsteps, and the ever-changing composition of colors and shapes that danced across my field of vision. This mindful engagement with the act of walking introduced a richness and depth to each moment I had never experienced so consciously, transforming a mundane activity into a deeply meditative and nourishing practice.

Since that garden visit, mindful walking has become a cherished part of my daily routine, a practice I carry with me wherever I go. Whether I find myself strolling through the quiet serenity of a wooded setting or a bustling city street, I know that this simple technique will readily ground me firmly in the present moment, gently muting the otherwise relentless tide of thoughts and distractions.

In a nutshell, mindful walking is the art of engaging fully with the act of walking, paying close attention to the sensations and experiences that accompany each step. This practice can be performed in a variety of settings, from the serenity of nature to the bustling streets of the urban jungle, offering a versatile and accessible means of cultivating mindfulness within our busy daily lives.

So I invite you to explore the re-engaging potential of mindful walking in your own life. By intentionally walking and immersing yourself in the myriad sensations and experiences that accompany your journey, you may find that this practice serves as a powerful tool for cultivating mindfulness, presence, and reinvigorating connection with the world around you.

④ Loving-Kindness Meditation

Rather than being a practice that was once unfamiliar to you or I, loving-kindness meditation is, in fact, the simple ritualization of doing what we do quite naturally with our loved ones, but more broadly and with greater frequency and intention.

Designed to bring us closer to one another and to our innermost selves, this is a practice that involves directing feelings of love, compassion, and goodwill toward ourselves and others. By focusing our attention on these positive emotions, we can cultivate a greater sense of connection and empathy, fostering a deep understanding of presence and engagement with the present moment.

To paint a clearer picture, I can draw upon the memory of an early pursuit of making this practice habit. I settled into a quiet space, dimly lit by the flickering glow of a solitary candle, and closed my eyes. As I inhaled deeply, I began to visualize myself as the recipient of my own love and compassion, directing these tender sentiments toward the person I knew best: myself.

As I progressed through the meditation, I expanded the sphere of my loving attention, gradually encompassing friends and family, acquaintances, and even those with whom I had experienced conflict or discord. At that moment, I recognized the universality of our human desire for love and connection, a truth that transcended the petty grievances and perceived slights that so often divide us.

As you embark upon your journey of loving-kindness meditation, you will probably be able to approach each interaction and encounter with a newfound sense of compassion and empathy, engaging more fully and opening your heart to the transformative power of love and compassion. By cultivating these qualities within ourselves, we can forge deeper connections with others and a greater sense of presence in the now.

❺ **Mindful Eating**

By now, you will no doubt have noticed an obvious pattern emerging—namely, the power of our senses to guide our minds back into our bodies and the present moment whenever we find ourselves cast adrift in the past or future.

As is the case with mindful walking, with a bit of thought, we discover other opportunities to harness our senses in a heightened state of engagement throughout the day. One such opportunity is during mealtimes, and the technique we can employ is mindful eating.

The practice of mindful eating involves engaging fully with the experience of eating, savoring the flavors, textures, and sensations of our food with deliberate and focused attention. This technique not only fosters a greater appreciation for the nourishment we receive but also serves to ground our awareness in the present moment, reinventing the mundane act of eating as a meditative and intentional experience.

> **Given that nourishment is such an essential part of the human experience, many may find this one of the easiest mindfulness techniques to try first. With that in mind, consider its power next time you sit down to dine and allow your senses to do the work of soothing and quieting your mind on your behalf.**

X.

The Long-Term Benefits of Mindfulness

The remarkable efficacy of mindfulness extends far beyond the fleeting moments of tranquility and presence it bestows upon us in a momentary practice. With consistent and dedicated practice, mindfulness can yield a spectrum of long-term benefits, fostering emotional well-being and catalyzing personal growth in profound and lasting ways.

In this chapter, we will explore how mindfulness can enrich our lives over time, leaving a lasting impact on our emotional health, relationships, and personal development.

① Cultivating Emotional Resilience

The journey of life, rife with its countless vicissitudes, is a testament to the impermanence of our worldly existence. Amidst the unceasing undercurrents of our daily experiences, emotional resilience emerges as a lighthouse in the distance, guiding us toward a sense of inner equanimity and stability.

As you have seen, my odyssey toward emotional resilience began with the simple yet profound practice of mindfulness. However, as I made mindfulness a constant companion through practice, I discovered that, once again, it was a stepping stone that raised another before it as I claimed the power of non-judgmental awareness.

By observing my thoughts and emotions with detached curiosity, I found myself better equipped to explore my inner world, embracing both light and shadow with equal acceptance.

I learned we could develop emotional resilience by embracing the unwelcome aspects of our human experience with open-hearted vulnerability instead of denying or suppressing them. As I grappled with my own fears, insecurities, and doubts, I gradually understood that these challenges were the catalysts for my growth, molding me into a stronger, more compassionate individual.

One salient instance that vividly encapsulates this journey toward resilience occurred during a particularly turbulent period of my life. Beset by a veritable maelstrom of professional and personal upheaval, I found myself teetering on the brink of despair.

Yet, in this darkest hour, the budding fruits of my mindfulness practice began to blossom. As I turned my gaze inward, I discovered a wellspring of inner strength, a quiet, unwavering resolve that allowed me to weather the storm and emerge stronger and more resilient on the other side than ever.

In retrospect, I now realize that it was through a wide-angled perspective on such adversity that I honed my emotional resilience. By cultivating a non-judgmental awareness of my thoughts and emotions, I developed the ability to respond with greater adaptability and flexibility.

As I reflect upon the granular details of my journey, I realize that emotional resilience is not an innate quality reserved for a few but rather a skill that anyone can develop and strengthen through consistent practice. In sharing this, I hope to inspire you to embark upon your own journey of self-discovery and embrace the transformative power of mindfulness for cultivating emotional resilience.

② Enhancing Self-Awareness and Personal Insight

My quest for self-awareness and personal insight has led me down a winding and uneven path, replete with moments of revelation and discovery. In the beginning, I was naught but a stranger to myself; the incessant chatter of my mind obscured my innermost thoughts and desires.

Only through my encounter with mindfulness did I find the cross marking the treasure trove of self-awareness that lay hidden within. As I uncovered my prize, gradually peeling back the layers of my psyche, I revealed areas of my inner world that were previously unknown.

By confronting the fears, insecurities, and doubts I had once subconsciously buried, I unearthed the deeply ingrained patterns and habits that had shaped my thoughts, emotions, and behaviors for so long. With each passing day, I became more attuned to the subtle nuances of my inner landscape, developing a heightened sensitivity to the ebb and flow of my mental and emotional currents.

In my pursuit of self-awareness, I found solace in the confessional, often intimate journaling process. Through the written word, I chronicled the minutia of my inner world, crafting an outward representation of the thoughts, emotions, and experiences that mirror my soul.

As I reflected upon the pages of my journal, I began to discern the patterns and themes that governed my life, gaining a deeper understanding of the forces that shape my identity and direction. In this way, through a practice of mindfulness-based journaling, we can each cultivate a heightened sense of self-awareness and personal insight, empowering us to recognize areas in need of growth and improvement.

③ Fostering Empathy and Compassion

On my journey toward the words that mark these pages, I have found empathy and compassion to be indispensable resources for strengthening relationships and fueling personal growth. I want to share with you, dear reader, the intimate details of my experiences cultivating these qualities in the hope that they may inspire you to explore this path as well.

My voyage into the realm of empathy and compassion began with a habitual practice of mindfulness. As I started practicing mindfulness, I focused on my inner world and faced my own suffering - the various emotions and fears that had been suppressed in my consciousness for a long time. In bearing witness to my pain, I developed a more profound sense of understanding and compassion for myself.

As I continued to traverse my inner world, I discovered, as many have before me, that my newfound compassion for myself had given rise to an increased sensitivity to the suffering of others.

The walls that had once separated me from those around me began to crumble, revealing the common thread of humanity that binds us all. I found myself more attuned to the emotional currents of others, able to discern their joys and sorrows with greater clarity and nuance.

In my efforts to foster empathy and compassion, I frequently returned to the confessional and intimate practice of loving-kindness meditation. With each heartfelt recitation of well-wishes for myself and others, I felt my capacity for empathy and compassion expand, enveloping all those with whom I crossed paths. As my heart opened, I found that my connections with others warmed and deepened.

My exploration of empathy and compassion has not been without its challenges. At times, I have been confronted with the overwhelming pain of others, a torrent of emotions that threatened to engulf me. Yet, through the practice of mindfulness, I have learned to approach such turbulence with kind acceptance; to remain grounded in the present moment and anchored in the strength that true presence provides.

Mindful of its benefits, I urge you to embark on your own quest for empathy and compassion. Through mindfulness and loving-kindness meditation, you can cultivate an open-hearted awareness of your own suffering and that of others, forging more meaningful and authentic connections with the people in your life.

May you find solace and inspiration in the knowledge that we are all connected by the common thread of humanity, bound together by our shared joys, successes, missteps, sorrows, and dreams.

④ Reducing Stress and Anxiety

Within the modern world, we each inevitably face our fair share of stress and anxiety. If I may, I'd like to share with you how mindfulness can be applied to reduce these debilitating emotions and reclaim a sense of inner peace.

During a trying time of looming deadlines, I came to appreciate the capacity of mindfulness to turn down the volume of stress and anxiety just as they may otherwise have run riot. With each deliberate breath, I began to anchor myself in the present moment, learning to observe the tempest of thoughts and emotions that raged within me without being swept into their forces.

By stepping briefly from my work to indulge in my daily mindfulness practice, I cultivated the ability to stand as a silent witness to my inner turmoil, observing my fears and anxieties as they arose and dissipated like passing clouds in the sky. I discerned the impermanent nature of these emotions, recognizing that they were but fleeting visitors in the vast expanse of my consciousness.

As I honed this skill, I found that my anxiety and stress waned, their grip on my mind and heart loosening as I learned to observe them without judgment or resistance. Slowly but surely, a sense of ease took root within me, allowing my productive mind to flow freely and without obstacles.

Many scientific studies have shown the efficacy of mindfulness in reducing stress and anxiety. By observing our thoughts and emotions without becoming entangled in them, we can meet the tensions and pressures of daily life without allowing an unhelpful reactionary inner response to take the reins.

⑤ Promoting a Growth Mindset

Like any author, I have experienced the peaks and valleys of a creative life, with both triumphs and setbacks. I remember a time when my writing fell stagnant, my inspiration dwindling as the wellspring of my creativity seemed to run dry.

I met each attempt to put pen to paper with resistance, and I spiraled into self-doubt and frustration. It was in this state of creative crisis that I turned to mindfulness as a means to invigorate the growth mindset that would reawaken my inner resources.

In the quiet moments of my practice, I noticed the patterns of self-judgment and criticism that had taken hold, preventing me from fully embracing the potential for growth that lay waiting for an opportunity to emerge.

As I cultivated a non-judgmental awareness of the unhelpful nature of this self-critical pattern of thought, I started to see my setbacks not as signs of failure but as opportunities for learning and development. Each challenge became a step on a ladder, guiding me upward toward a more intuitive connection between my craft and myself.

I found myself approaching my writing with a renewed sense of curiosity and wonder, embracing the unknown with an open heart and mind. I began viewing my creative process as a journey of continuous growth and discovery, a voyage into uncharted territory with infinite potential for transformation and self-improvement.

With each mindful breath taken at my desk, I cultivated the resilience and adaptability necessary to face adversity head-on, fostering a growth mindset that transformed my relationship with my art and myself. No longer did I shy away from the challenges that arose; instead, I saw them as invitations to delve deeper, learn, and grow.

> **I hope that this may inspire you to explore the vast potential for learning and development that lies within your own life. Embrace the obstacles you encounter with curiosity and wonder, and you will find that each challenge becomes a rung on an upward journey of personal growth and self-discovery.**

XI.

A Cautionary Tale of Hubris and Ignorance

In the grand theatre of human emotions and behaviors, few traits are as deceptively simplistic and yet as insidiously destructive as arrogance. Often cloaked in a veil of confidence and self-assuredness, arrogance belies a more sinister nature, one that can lead to profound consequences for both the individual and those around them.

In this chapter, we shall delve into the beguiling simplicity of arrogance, exploring its subtle manifestations and the far-reaching impact it can have on our lives and the lives of others.

Arrogance is rooted in the misguided belief in one's infallibility, with an inflated sense of self-importance and an overestimation of one's abilities, talents, or knowledge. It is this misguided belief in one's infallibility that lies at the heart of arrogance's trap.

For the arrogant individual, they view the world through a distorted lens that magnifies their own perceived greatness while diminishing the value and worth of others. In this warped reality, they reduce the complexities and nuances of the world to a mere backdrop against which their own superiority takes center stage.

The consequences of arrogance are manifold, and their impact can reverberate far beyond the confines of the individual's life. Arrogance in interpersonal relationships generates discord and resentment as the arrogant individual's self-aggrandizing behavior makes others feel inferior or dismissed. Friendships are strained, and it weakens bonds as the arrogant person becomes increasingly isolated in their own self-imposed fortress of ego and self-righteousness.

In the professional sphere, arrogance can prove to be a formidable obstacle to success and growth. The arrogant individual's inability to recognize their own limitations and shortcomings often leads to poor decision-making and a failure to learn from mistakes. Their inflated sense of self-importance can also hinder collaboration and teamwork as they struggle to accept input and constructive criticism from their colleagues.

Arrogance can have a corrosive effect on personal growth and self-improvement. By refusing to acknowledge their flaws and imperfections, the arrogant individual effectively stifles their development, stagnating in a quagmire of self-deception and hubris. In this state, growth becomes an elusive and unattainable goal, as the individual remains not blissfully but frustratedly ignorant of their shortcomings and life lessons.

> **By cultivating humility, curiosity, and empathy, we can counteract the insidious influence of arrogance in our lives, fostering a more open-minded, compassionate, and growth-oriented existence. In this way, we can unravel the tangled web of ego and self-deception, creating a more authentic, meaningful, and fulfilling life for ourselves and those around us.**

XII.

Deconstructing the Breathtaking Assumption of Linear Time

The inexorable march of time is a constant and unyielding force, propelling us through the vast expanse of human experience with relentless determination. Yet, in our quest to comprehend the enigma of time, we often fall prey to a breathtaking assumption: that we can strip a moment in time of its infinite complexity and reduce it to a mere sequence of linear events.

In this chapter, we shall endeavor to deconstruct this beguiling assumption, examining the byzantine miscellany of moments that comprise our existence and the subtle nuances that render each moment a microcosm of infinite complexity.

The allure of linear time is undeniable, offering us a semblance of order and predictability amidst the chaos of our lives. We quantify our days by the clock's ticking, our routines and rituals dictated by the steady progression of hours, minutes, and seconds.

Yet, beneath this veneer of simplicity lies a rich and intricate web of interconnected moments, each serving as a unique and widely networked junction channeling emotions, experiences, and perceptions.

To truly appreciate the infinite complexity of a moment in time, we must slide beneath the surface of linear progression and examine the many factors that converge to shape our experience of each moment. The unfolding present creates a kaleidoscope of experiential touchpoints that defy any attempt at reduction or simplification. The unfolding present and our thoughts, emotions, and sensory perceptions are inextricably intertwined.

Furthermore, the very nature of time itself is a subject of profound debate and speculation among philosophers, physicists, and scholars alike. From the eternalism of the block universe theory to the fleeting ephemerality of the presentism view, the concept of time has been the subject of countless theories and conjectures throughout the ages. In this context, we can strip the assumption that a moment in time of its complexity becomes even more tenuous and ill-founded.

The consequences of this breathtaking assumption are far-reaching and significant. By reducing our experience of time to a mere sequence of linear events, we risk losing sight of additions to the ever-shifting and growing pattern of moments that make up our lives.

In doing so, we may become so preoccupied with the past and future that we fail to fully engage with the present, missing out on the richness and depth of experience that can only be found in the here and now.

> **By cultivating a deeper appreciation for the subtleties and nuances that define and enrich our existence, we can begin to unravel the fruitless assumption of linear time, forging a more authentic, meaningful, and expansive understanding of our ever-unfolding realities.**

XIII.

Confronting Our Dislike for Unforeseen Outcomes

In our ceaseless pursuit of personal fulfillment and success, we often find ourselves clinging to a rigid set of expectations, meticulously crafting visions of how we believe our lives should unfold. Yet, as we navigate the unpredictable currents of human existence, something invariably confronts us with outcomes that fail to align with these carefully constructed blueprints.

In this chapter, we shall confront our disquiet when such outcomes arrive, examining the roots of our discontent and the liberating potential that lies within the acceptance of the unexpected.

At the core of our aversion to the unforeseen lies a fundamental human desire for control, an innate longing to impose order and predictability upon the chaotic nature of our lives. We strive to chart a course through the murky waters of uncertainty, seeking comfort in the illusion of control that our expectations provide. When the tides of life fail to heed our well-laid plans, we are left grappling with disappointment, our vision of the world suddenly thrown into disarray.

This dislikes for outcomes that defy our expectations is further compounded by the weight of societal norms and pressures, which dictate the benchmarks by which we measure our success and self-worth. When our lives can not align with these prescribed ideals, we may experience feelings of inadequacy and failure. The discord between our expectations and reality may threaten our sense of identity and self-esteem.

Yet, within our discontent lies the very ingredients for transformation and growth. By confronting our animosity toward unforeseen outcomes, we can unravel the tightly woven expectations and desire for control that bind us, cultivating a greater capacity for adaptability, resilience, and acceptance in the face of life's inherent unpredictability.

The key to navigating the chasm between our expectations and reality lies in embracing the wisdom of uncertainty and recognizing the futility of attempting to impose order upon the inherently chaotic nature of existence. By relinquishing our attachment to specific outcomes, we can learn to find meaning and even joy as the steps of life's dance continue to change.

In this pursuit of acceptance, we may also find ourselves better equipped to identify and appreciate the hidden gifts and lessons that unforeseen outcomes can bring, for it is often in the unexpected twists and turns of life's journey that we encounter the most charged opportunities for growth, self-discovery, and transformation.

> **So, as we move forward, let us strive to confront the clarity of our dislike for unforeseen outcomes, acknowledge the limitations of our expectations, and embrace the liberating potential of uncertainty. In this way, we can forge a more authentic, adaptive, and expansive existence, one that is guided by the wisdom of experience rather than the narrow confines of expectation and control.**

XIV.
Leveraging Acceptance to Reconcile the Past and the Present

As we push forward across life's hills and valleys, we are often confronted with the specters of the past, shadowy echoes of regret, resentment, and longing that cling to the recesses of our consciousness. In this chapter, we shall examine the healing power of acceptance, exploring its vital role in reconciling the past with the potential of the present moment.

At its core, acceptance is an act of profound surrender, a relinquishing of the futile quest to control and manipulate the immutable nature of what has gone before the now. It is the recognition that, while we cannot change what has transpired, we possess the power to shape our perception of these events and, in doing so, transform how they inform our present experience.

In reconciling with the past, we must first acknowledge the complete and complex color scape of our emotions, memories, and experiences as they define our personal histories. To reconcile with the past, we need to muster courage and vulnerability to confront the scars and wounds that are etched upon the canvas of our souls during introspection. Only through this honest examination of our past can we begin to prime a clear surface for the acceptance and healing we wish to paint.

The embrace of acceptance allows us to view our past through the lens of compassion and understanding, recognizing the lessons and growth that have emerged from even the most painful of experiences. By accepting the past for what it is, we can release the burdens of regret, bitterness, and self-recrimination that have weighed us down, liberating ourselves from the shackles of resentment and blame.

Simultaneously, acceptance empowers us to seize the present moment, unencumbered by the ghosts of our past. As we learn to accept life's inherent unpredictability and impermanence, we become better prepared to maneuver within the present, cultivating a sense of groundedness and presence that allows us to fully and authentically engage.

> **With this framing, as we continue our exploration of the human condition, let us strive to cultivate a deeper sense of acceptance and letting go, recognizing the freeing possibility that emerges when we reconcile with the past and embrace the present. In doing so, we will find not only healing but also a more expansive, fulfilling, and harmonious existence.**

XV.

The Alchemy of Acceptance and Unburdening the Soul

Most people have experienced the discomfort of needing to cultivate acceptance and release the burdens of the past that weigh upon their hearts, whether knowingly or unknowingly. In this chapter, we shall take a tour through some practical strategies for embracing acceptance, unlocking a series of tangible tools and techniques that can aid us in our quest to unburden the soul and foster a more profound sense of inner harmony and peace.

① **Mindful Reflection:**

In the whirlwind of life's continued momentum, we can meet the cascade of our thoughts and emotions, so often roaring like the ephemeral notes of a symphony, with the practice of mindful reflection. Serving as a demonstration of this technique, I remember one particularly poignant evening as I sat beside the warmth of a flickering fire, its light casting an amber glow upon the room.

I found myself lost in the maze of my memories, each one laden with the weight of emotion and expectation. At this moment, I consciously approached these recollections with the same grace and acceptance that I had cultivated through my mindfulness practice.

As I turned my attention to untangling these thoughts, I began examining my past events and experiences with a newfound sense of curiosity and compassion. The triumphs and tribulations, the joys and sorrows, each moment presented itself to me as an essential sum part of my life's valuable wholeness.

In the stillness of that quiet night, I felt a profound sense of connection to the totality of my being, as though I had, for the first time, embraced the full spectrum of my humanity. This mindful reflection illuminated and continues to illuminate the path of my personal journey, growing with each revisit and revealing the inherent beauty and purpose that lies within each moment.

To begin your mindful reflection, the first step is to allow yourself to become fully present with the medley of thoughts, emotions, and sensations that comprise your unique narrative. By cultivating acceptance, you can also discover the transformative power of mindful reflection. You can find within the depths of your past an inviting pool of self-compassion that you can always return to.

② **Expressive Writing:**

In the quiet solitude of my study, I have found refuge in the act of expressive writing, an endeavor that has proven to be a powerful instrument for healing and transformation. With each stroke of the pen, it has granted me passage into the uncharted depths of my soul, uncovering the hidden facets of my inner landscape that have long eluded me.

I recall an evening not long ago when the weight of the world seemed to rest squarely on my shoulders. My thoughts were a tempestuous sea, churning with a relentless barrage of emotions, each wave crashing upon the shores of my consciousness with unyielding force. At this moment, I turned not to the solace of my journal but to the clean page of a new notebook where I could unleash my imagination.

As I began to pour experimental thoughts and feelings onto the page, I found that, quite counterintuitively, the act of writing imaginatively served to anchor me in the present moment, providing an abstract space in which to explore the tangles of my mind safely.

With each word that flowed from my pen, I felt as though I was unraveling the threads of my past, gaining insight and understanding into the myriad factors that had shaped my perspective of the world and informed my present experience.

The process of expressive writing revealed to me the beauty and power of vulnerability, allowing me to confront my fears, insecurities, and doubts with honesty and courage. In bearing witness to my truth, I found I was able to release the burdens of regret and shame that had long had me locked in their vice-like grip.

So with great humility, I encourage you to commit your thoughts and imaginings to paper. You will surely unleash a potent catalyst for non-judgmental growth as you place your own exploratory thoughts and feelings on the page.

❸ Forgiveness

In the quiet recesses of my heart, I have found that the need for forgiveness often punctuates the journey toward acceptance. It is an arduous task, one that requires us to confront the corners of our past and face the pain and heartache that has arisen from the actions of both ourselves and others.

In the sanctity of my study, I understand that forgiveness is not merely an act of absolution but rather a transformative process that fosters empathy, understanding, and, ultimately, healing.

In doing so, I recalled a time when I found myself shackled by the chains of resentment, the bitter sting of betrayal lingering long after the events that had transpired. As I sat with my thoughts, consumed by the anguish of a wounded heart, I came to realize that the path to redemption lay not in retribution but in forgiveness.

In the ensuing days, I embarked upon a journey of introspection. I realized we are all, in our own ways, imperfect beings, navigating the stormy waters of existence with only the tools and resources we have at our disposal.

In cultivating an understanding of the shared humanity that connects us all, I saw the events of my past through the lens of empathy and compassion, recognizing the interplay of forces that had given rise to the perceived wrongs and transgressions that had caused me pain. It was then that I found the strength to forgive not only those who had wronged me but also myself for my role in unfolding events.

The need to forgive both ourselves and others for the perceived wrongs and transgressions that have caused us pain often marks the journey toward acceptance.

As you consider when to plunge into the depths of your heart in search of the unforgiven, may you find the courage to embrace empathy and understanding, recognizing the inherent imperfections that define our existence and the shared humanity that connects us all.

④ Gratitude

As I recline in my favorite armchair, a warm cup of tea cradled in my hands, I am reminded of the gentle power of gratitude. It is a practice that has served as a candle, awakening and cleansing the darker recesses of my existence, guiding me toward a place of acceptance and peace.

In these quiet moments of modest solitude, I have come to understand how gratitude invites us to shift our gaze from the disappointments and regrets of the past to the abundance and beauty that lies within the present moment.

Through the practice of gratitude, I have also learned to view life's events not as a series of discrete occurrences but rather as a cohesive narrative.

With each addition to this inner library, I am reminded of the countless reasons I have to be grateful, from the richness of my relationships to the bountiful beauty of the natural world that surrounds me.

Through this practice, I view the events of my past not as obstacles to be overcome but as opportunities for growth and transformation. In embracing gratitude, I have found a newfound sense of acceptance and peace, one that transcends the transitory nature of my experiences and anchors me firmly within the present moment.

Consider this a calling to explore the practice of gratitude in your own life. As you reflect upon the merry band of experiences that have shaped your journey, may you be courageous, cultivating a sense of gratitude for the lessons and growth that have emerged and, in doing so, fostering the tranquility that only gratitude can provide.

⑤ Releasing Rituals

One starry autumn evening, I found myself seated at my writing desk, pouring forth the burdens of my past, the pain, and sorrow that have clung to the corners of my heart, as I crafted a letter to the person I once was. This intimate act of confession, borne from the depths of my soul, served as a symbolic gesture, a means of releasing the shackles that have bound me to the past.

Inscribed within the lines of this letter were the recriminations that have haunted me; each word impressed not only with pigment but with the weight of an unspoken emotion. As the ink dried upon the page, I felt a sense of liberation wash over me, as though the act of committing these thoughts to paper had somehow loosened their grip upon my spirit.

With the letter now complete, I made my way to the garden, the earth beneath my feet cool and damp as I trod lightly among the slumbering flowers. In the darkness, I dug a small hole, a resting place for my heartfelt missive, a vessel in which to release the past. As I buried the letter, I performed a quiet ceremony, a whispered invocation to the forces of nature, the elements that have borne witness to the unfolding of my life.

This simple act of ritualized release, the symbolic burial of my past burdens, serves as a powerful catalyst for transformation and healing. It is a sacred rite of passage, one that has allowed me to step more fully into the present moment, unencumbered by the weight of past regrets and sorrows.

Engaging in rituals and ceremonies designed to facilitate the release of past burdens can be a powerful means of fostering acceptance and letting go. Such rituals may take the form of symbolic acts, such as writing a letter to one's past self or creating a visual representation of the burdens we wish to release, followed by a ceremonial act of release, such as burning or burying the symbolic artifact.

I encourage you to experiment boldly with the power of releasing rituals in your own life, seeking the symbolic act of ceremonial release that resonates most with you. In doing so, you may find a newfound sense of freedom and acceptance, a lightness of being that accompanies the shedding of past burdens.

⑥ Seeking Support

All who have stood upon the precipice of change, the winds of uncertainty whipping about them, will have found themselves beset by a profound sense of vulnerability, their hearts laid bare to the tempestuous emotions that, in such moments, churn within.

It was during one of these very moments of self-doubt and trepidation that I came to understand the immeasurable value of seeking support from those who had walked the path before me.

With a tentative step, I reached out to those I trusted most, my confidantes and allies in this journey toward acceptance and healing. Through our intimate exchanges, I discovered that guidance could be a balm for the wounds that our souls bear. Friends, family, and mental health professionals can offer wisdom and compassion to help reform our strength and courage when facing demons.

It is a curious thing, this act of seeking support, for in the vulnerability of our confessions, we find a strength that transcends the limits of our individual selves. We become part of something greater, a collective consciousness that carries both the weight of our burdens and us forward, one step at a time.

May this idea spur you to embrace this transformative power of connection to seek the support of those who can guide and accompany you on your journey toward healing and self-discovery. In seeking the support of allies, we can find solace and guidance as we progress, so let us endeavor to incorporate these practical strategies and the alchemy of acceptance into our daily lives.

XVI.

The Elixir and Rewards of Acceptance

In our ongoing exploration of the transformative power of acceptance, we have traversed the landscape of practical strategies and mindful approaches that can aid us in releasing the burdens of the past and embracing the present moment.

In this chapter, we shall turn our gaze toward the manifold benefits of acceptance for personal and emotional development, examining how this potent elixir can nourish the soul and catalyze growth.

(1) Cultivating Inner Peace

A key chapter of my voyage on the ship of acceptance involved a deliberate journey into calmer waters. To release my attachment to the narratives that had long held me within swirling surges, I had to steer understanding that I could not rewrite the past or alter the course of events that had shaped me.

With each unfamiliar leg of progress, I felt the weight of my self-imposed anchorage lessen, the burden of my suffering and discontent easing as I relinquished the rope that had rigidly moored me to the past.

Armed with this newfound approach, I soon sailed into a sanctuary of solace, a place within myself where the restless waters of my soul began to calm. As I floated upon the mirror-like surface of this haven, the stillness increasingly radiated outward from my mighty vessel, and a sense of peace arose that moved through every fiber of my being.

The practice of acceptance invites you, just as it did me, to find your own calm inner waters as you release your attachment to the narratives and judgments that cloud your perception of the past and steer, knowing that you cannot change what has transpired.

As you master releasing your own anchor chains of regret and resentment, you can foster a more profound sense of inner peace, freeing yourself from the fetters of suffering and discontent.

② **Enhancing Resilience**

On the next stage of my journey, as I strolled along the shores of my existence, the sands shifting beneath my feet with each passing tide, I began to focus my perception on the transient nature of life, the ephemeral dance of change that plays out in every facet of our being. From the rhythmic beating of our hearts to the ceaseless procession of the seasons, life's most reliable facets are impermanence and unpredictability.

Upon this realization, I discovered the potential for resilience that lay within me, a strength forged alongside my experiences and tempered by my willingness to embrace the undulating sands of being. I found contentedness in the knowledge that nothing is constant and that each moment, no matter how fleeting or seemingly insignificant, lays out endless avenues of possibility for us to explore.

Crucially, in learning to accept the mystery of our future, we can become more adept at navigating circumstances and charting a course through adversity with a fresh sense of resilience and adaptability.

No longer must we fear the winds of change, but rather, we can embrace them as opportunities for growth, as stimulation for the evolution of the soul. By embracing the inherent vacillations of life, we cultivate a greater capacity to weather the changeable dune-scape of adversity and change.

③ Promoting Emotional Healing

As we have discovered, the healing process requires not only introspection but also the cultivation of compassion, empathy, and self-acceptance. To provide a sense of what this looks like, it was in the quiet, candlelit corners of my soul that I began unraveling the threads of my past gently, allowing the light of awareness to brighten the role that they play within my emotional tapestry.

With each tender stitch I traced, my comprehension of the connections that define consciousness grew. I learned to cradle my wounded heart in the soft embrace of understanding, to hold my pain with the tender touch of compassion, and to forgive myself for the moments of weakness and despair that had punctuated my past.

In time, the wounds that I once personified began to fade, replaced by the verdant hues of emotional growth and transformation. As I liberated myself from the bonds of my past traumas, healing that had once seemed unattainable quickly picked up its pace.

The journey toward acceptance often necessitates the exploration of the wounds and scars that linger within our emotional landscape. As we engage in this process of introspection and healing, we pave the way for emotional growth and transformation, so I invite you to turn courage and compassion inward in the knowledge that they are powerful salves for gently lifting the scars of life.

④ Fostering Self-Compassion

Of course, to harness compassion, we must first know how to ignite it. So I recall, dear reader, a time when I peered, unequipped, into the deep of my past with a mixture of trepidation and curiosity. From this bird's-eye perspective, I could see that the fog of judgment and self-criticism had clouded my perception of my past. It was as if I had been viewing my own story through a distorted lens.

Not yet ready to descend, with each downward, I endeavored to soften my gaze and view my past with the gentle, loving eyes of compassion and understanding. I sought to recognize the inherent beauty and wisdom that lay within each of my experiences, to honor the many lessons that had been imparted to me in the forming of each memory.

In time, I discovered that self-compassion cultivation was akin to tending a delicate, blossoming flower that required the nourishment of love, empathy, and understanding to flourish. As I nurtured this tender bloom, I found that my relationship with myself began to transcend, unfurling into a loving and compassionate bond with the self so powerful that I could plumb the depths of my past without losing my thread to the present.

To view your own story with the gentle, loving eyes of understanding and empathy, all that is required is to practice the art of self-compassion until it becomes second nature.

In accepting the past for what it is, we can begin to view our personal histories through the lens of kindness and understanding. This shift in perspective allows us to cultivate a more loving and empathetic relationship with ourselves, which alters our relationships with others.

⑤ Unlocking Personal Growth

A secret trove of wisdom and growth exists that lies deep within the recesses of our past. As I pondered this notion, I found myself drawn to exploring my history, seeking to unearth the pearls of insight that lay nestled amongst the debris of my trials and tribulations.

At first, the prospect of delving into the darker corners of my memory was daunting, fraught with the specter of old hurts and regrets that threatened to engulf me in their obscuring embrace. Yet, as I ventured further into the labyrinth of my past, I began to perceive the faint glimmers of understanding that shone upward through the gloom, signposting the unseen worth of events and experiences that had shaped my life.

In time, I recognized the transformative potential that lay hidden within even the most painful of memories. I learned to see the beauty in the struggle, the wisdom in the wound, and the strength in the scar. This newfound perspective allowed me to view my past not as a burden to be borne but as fertile soil from which the seeds of personal growth and self-discovery could take root and flourish.

Acceptance invites us to conquer the hidden recesses of our past, unearthing the lessons and wisdom that lie beneath even the most painful experiences. As you learn to recognize and embrace that which is hidden, you will discover your fertile trove and give root to the authentic, expansive, and fulfilling existence that bursts forth with personal growth.

 Strengthening Relationships

There is a certain beauty in cultivating acceptance within ourselves, a subtle chemistry that transmutes the leaden weight of our imperfections into the golden warmth of empathy and understanding. However, this alchemic art does not permeate only our relationship with the self. It can also transform the bonds we share with others.

To reference my own experience, in embracing the idiosyncrasies and imperfections that define our shared humanity, I strengthened the bonds of affection and understanding that connected me to my fellow travelers on this journey of life.

In fact, I recall precisely the period within which I began to see my loved ones not as flawed individuals but as fellow souls, each grappling with their unique tapestry of joys and sorrows, victories and defeats.

In that recognition, I found forgiveness and grace, a balm that soothed the rough edges of our interactions and fostered abundant harmony. As I continued cultivating this spirit of acceptance and understanding, I found that my relationships began to flourish. The barriers that once separated us began to dissolve, revealing a sense of intimacy and closeness built upon a foundation of mutual respect and appreciation.

> **As we cultivate acceptance within ourselves, we naturally become more open and understanding in our interactions with others. So probe the transformative potential of acceptance into your relationships. As you cultivate a deeper understanding of yourself and others, may you discover the beauty and strength within our shared imperfections, and may your relationships grow brightly under the gentle light of empathy, compassion, and mutual understanding.**

XVII.

The Eternal Present and Embracing the Moment

As we stand upon the threshold of the present, our gaze drawn inexorably toward the entrancing lights of the past and future, it is easy to become ensnared within that lingering neon glow, prone to cast its color upon our perception of the here and now.

Yet we can claim our true potential only within the bright clarity of the eternal present. So in this chapter, I will guide you toward familiarity with the importance of turning firmly into the present moment in readiness for the challenges and triumphs that life bestows upon us.

 The Illusory Nature of Time

Ah, the enigmatic nature of time. As we have already explored, time is a confounding construct that has entranced and intrigued the great minds of our species for millennia. Yet, as I have pondered this elusive entity, I have often found myself compelled to plunge into its very essence, to unravel the threads that pull us back and forth along the central strand of its inexorable march.

In my contemplations, I began to perceive more clearly that the past, present, and future coalesce into a singular dance, a fluid interplay of moments that appear and vanish like wisps of smoke upon the breeze.

This revelation soon guided me, perhaps surprisingly, not into distant eras but ever deeper into the present moment, allowing me to fully immerse myself in the richness that defines our existence.

In our quest to understand the significance of the present moment, it is imperative that we first acknowledge the illusory nature of time itself. Time, as we perceive it, is but a construct of the human mind, a linear progression of moments that exist solely within the realm of our consciousness.

By recognizing the inherent transience and impermanence of time, we can begin to free ourselves from its confining grasp, allowing us to embrace the eternal now fully.

As you discover the countless intersections that hold the power to dissolve the illusory nature of time in your own journey, recognizing the fleeting dance of moments that comprise the symphony of our lives, you will see that past and present realities are as changeable as the weather. In doing so, may you find liberation in the eternal now, and may your heart rejoice in the boundless expanse of the present moment, where all possibilities live.

② The Power of Presence

The present moment, that elusive, transient, and yet abundant point upon which our existence teeters, holds a power of immeasurable magnitude within its delicate embrace. As I ventured upon my journey of self-discovery, I became acutely aware of the profound significance of this ephemeral instant, a fleeting glimpse of an eternity that exists at the nexus of past and future.

As I have learned, the power of presence lies in the ability to harness the full extent of our thoughts, actions, and choices within the confines of this singular moment. It is within this sliver of time, this impermanent space, that we hold the keys to our destiny, the tools with which to sculpt our reality and forge the path that lies before us.

As I immerse myself in the present, I increasingly find that my experiences and the wisdom gleaned from them begin to coalesce, providing me with a serene sense of purpose. Guided by the steady hand of intention, I can craft the intricate tapestry of my life consciously, each decision and deed weaving yet another vibrant thread into the ever-evolving tableau of my existence.

Embracing the power of presence, dear reader is akin to stepping through the looking glass. The present moment, fleeting and temporary though it may be, is the only point in time in which we wield the power to shape our reality. It is through this conscious engagement with the here and now that we are granted the capacity to shape our reality, seize the reins of our destiny, and navigate the uncharted waters of our future with grace, purpose, and unyielding determination.

May you, too, discover the transformative power of presence within your own life, and may it serve as a guiding light upon your path, illuminating the way forward as you journey ever onward toward your highest aspirations and most cherished dreams.

 The Art of Surrender

Life often brings us face-to-face with the harsh reality of uncertainty and the turbulent tides of change. It is during these moments, as the storms of existence rage around us, that we find ourselves grasping for a semblance of control, a means by which to weather the maelstrom that threatens to consume us.

My journey, often touched by a desire to exert control over outcomes rather than simply steering with wisdom, has led me to the realization that there is an art to surrender, a delicate balance between action and acquiescence that holds the key to inner peace and equanimity.

As I have interpreted it, this art of surrender is not a form of passive resignation but rather a conscious choice to release our attachment to the outcomes and circumstances that lie beyond the scope of our capacity. It is a transaction with the rolling waves of existence, an embrace of the impermanence and unpredictability that pervade the ever-shifting realities of the time.

As I learned to relinquish my attempted grip on the future, I discovered that the present moment offered a peaceful place from which to consider my next endeavor. In surrendering to the unfolding of life, I found myself able to guide my trajectory in so far as my view forward would allow, not with a certainty of my destination but also no longer at the mercy of the storm.

In the face of life's many challenges, it is all too easy to become mired in the quagmire of worry, fear, and doubt. The art of surrender is a journey of self-discovery, a path that leads us into the heart of our existence and allows us to traverse the landscape of our lives with unshakable ease. So may you, too, find quiet confidence in the embrace of surrender and a lively interest in what may be about to appear on the horizon.

4. The Wisdom of Impermanence

Allow me, if you will, to share a truth unveiled to me as I've waded through life's periodic swamps. This axiom lies within the very essence of our existence, a hidden gem that gleams with the wisdom of impermanence.

As we each wander through the intersecting passages of time, it becomes increasingly clear that all we hold dear and cherish is destined to fade into the mists of memory. The sands of our lives slip through our fingers, their grains sparkling with the fleeting beauty of transient moments.

And yet, it is within this very impermanence, this adept tango of creation and dissolution, that we uncover the gift that only the transitory can bestow. Indeed, as we embrace the evanescent nature of our experiences, we awaken to the realization that every moment, no matter how brief or fleeting, holds within it a kernel of wisdom, a nugget of truth that serves to energize that which will follow.

As we gaze upon the unfolding panorama of our lives, it is only in recognizing its precious nature that we can claim a sense of awe and reverence for the transient dance of light and shadow that plays out before our very eyes. The present moment, ephemeral though it may be, becomes infused with a richness and depth that transcends the boundaries of time and space, elevating our experience of the world to new heights of understanding.

As we journey ever onward while trying to selectively pause the present moment, we are continually confronted with the instability and transience of all that we hold dear. So, I invite you to join me in this exploration of the wisdom of impermanence, to step through the veil of illusion that muddies our perception of the world, and to embrace the exquisite uniqueness of the present moment in time, made possible only by its fleeting nature.

5 The Dance of Life

Let us indulge together in learning a few new steps that may heighten your own dance of life. But before we do, I must ask that you take a moment to observe the exquisite and intricate interplay of light and shadow, joy and sorrow, triumph and defeat, that weaves itself through the very fabric of the human experience. For within this sacred dance lies the potential for growth, learning, and evolution, with each step met by a new doorway to transformation and awakening.

As your steps mimic mine and we spin in this eternal dance, we also witness the opposing forces that shape our every moment. It is within the swirling eddies of this cosmic choreography that we find our greatest opportunities for growth, and we learn to embrace the now in all its infinite complexity.

With each simple or flamboyant step we take upon this mortal coil, we are offered a choice: to resist the dance of life with our next step or surrender ourselves to its energetic lead.

As we learn to follow the movements of the present rather than repeating those of the past or trying to anticipate those of the future, we find ourselves more fully inhabiting our hearts and minds, attuned to the subtle melody of existence that plays out right here, between the distractions of our peripherals.

In a wholehearted embrace of the dance of life, we allow ourselves to be carried along on the currents of change and transformation, our emotional lungs expanding with each literal breath we take. We celebrate the beauty and wonder of our shared human journey, our souls resonating with the song of creation that echoes through the vast expanse of time and space.

So, dear reader, as we embark upon this short but potent sequence of steps together, let us rejoice in the eternal present, in the sacred dance of life that unites us all. Let us open ourselves to the beauty and wonder surrounding us, allowing us to be transformed and awakened by the exquisite tapestry of moments that comprise our existence.

> **For it is within this dance, this delicate interplay of light and shadow, that we discover the true essence of our being and the boundless potential that lies within each and every one of us.**

XVIII.

Navigating the Currents of Time With Mindful Anchors

As our vessels are tossed upon the waves of past and future, the practice of mindfulness emerges not as a drowning anchor but as one that we can raise and drop as we please, helping us to remain firmly in the present moment or navigate back to it whenever we accidentally cast ourselves adrift.

In this chapter, we shall consider how the practice of mindfulness can serve as a dynamic anchor as we navigate the currents of time.

① The Essence of Mindfulness

In a world that so often demands our unyielding attention, mindfulness offers us a restful haven of stillness and serenity where we can reconnect with our innermost selves. Through the gentle art of mindfulness, it encouraged us to explore our inner and outer worlds with curiosity, compassion, and openness, allowing the veil of illusion to fall away, revealing the boundless wonder that resides at our side within everyday awareness.

As we embark upon this journey of mindfulness, we find ourselves cultivating a greater sense of connection with ourselves and the world around us. With each breath, we take an opportunity to sink more deeply into the sacred present.

Once tumbling and anarchic, our minds begin to settle like the surface of a still pond, allowing us to sense the totality of our being while looking outward with clarity.

No longer swayed by the capricious winds of desire or aversion, we find ourselves more fully aligned with and receptive to our ever-unfolding existence. For it is in this sacred space of stillness and serenity, with the essence of mindfulness distilled, that we uncover the true nature of our being, a boundless expanse of love, wisdom, and interconnectedness.

At its core, mindfulness is the practice of cultivating present-moment awareness, a state of focused attention and non-judgmental observation that allows us to fully experience and appreciate the here and now.

So as we delve further into the practical aspects of mindfulness, let us be guided by the light of curiosity, compassion, and openness, allowing ourselves to become masters navigators of the practice, claiming all of the tranquility that is entailed.

② The Mindful Observer

Allow me to share with you a revelation of utmost importance, a cornerstone upon which we build the practice of mindfulness: the cultivation of the observer's mind. This state of detached awareness, a gentle and steadfast presence, enables us to bear witness to our thoughts, emotions, and sensations as they ebb and flow without becoming ensnared in their swirling currents.

As we embark upon this journey into the depths of our consciousness, we may find ourselves confronted by a coalescence of thoughts and emotions clamoring for our attention like unruly children. Yet, in the cultivation of the observer's mind, we discover the capacity to remain unswayed by these capricious forces, our gaze unwavering and serene, like a lighthouse guiding our consciousness through the storm.

As we develop this ability to observe our inner landscape with aplomb, we create a space for insight and understanding, a sanctuary where the seeds of wisdom can take root and flourish. With each moment of mindful observation, we learn to interpret the events of our lives with greater grace and discernment, our steps guided by the light of our own innate wisdom.

In this sacred space of detached awareness, we find ourselves more fully attuned to the present moment, our senses alive and receptive to the boundless marvels that surround us. As a result, our hearts are expansive, and we can embrace the full spectrum of human experience, the joys, and sorrows, the triumphs and defeats, each moment an opportunity to become a greater version of the self.

And so, I encourage you to cultivate the observer's mind and forge conduits to the wisdom that lies within. For it is in the practice of mindfulness that we not only witness our thoughts, emotions, and sensations as they arise but choose whether they have a role to play in our ongoing evolution.

③ **Breathing as an Anchor**

Having already introduced you to the most humble yet remarkably transformative cornerstone of mindfulness practice, the breath, we will continue our journey toward fully understanding its value. This constant companion, ever-present and unyielding, serves as a ready anchor for our wandering minds, guiding us back to the sanctuary of the present moment time and time again.

As we embark upon self-exploration, we may find ourselves adrift in the turbulent seas of thought and emotion. The relentless tides of daily life pull our minds hither and thither. Yet, in the simple act of attending to our breath, we find a calm opening that leads us back to the here and now, where we can regain our footing and reconnect with all that truly matters.

With each inhalation and exhalation, it invited us to anchor more deeply into the present moment, our awareness attuned to the gentle rise and fall of our chest, the cool air caressing our nostrils, and the subtle sensations accompanying each breath. In this sacred space of focused attention, we cultivate a deep sense of connection to our own bodies and the world around us, fostering a sense of groundedness, stability, and peace.

As we move through the ever-changing landscape of our lives, the breath is a constant reminder of our innate capacity for presence and tranquility, a beacon of light that can guide us through the darkest of nights and the stormiest of seas. By repeatedly focusing on our breath, we can rediscover our innate ability to be present and joyful. This will open our hearts and minds to the endless possibilities that lie before us.

Knowing this, I urge you to embrace the power of the breath, to allow its gentle cadence to guide you back to the present moment whenever you need a guide, for it is within the inward and outward flow of our breath that we find the key to a more grounded, stable, and peaceful existence, anchored with intention in the eternal now.

④ Embodied Awareness

It is my humble pleasure to acquaint you with an aspect of mindfulness that is often overshadowed by the exploration of our thoughts and emotions: the realm of embodied awareness.

As we begin the work of consciously weaving the intricate tapestry of our lives, it offers us a unique opportunity to delve into the rich landscape of our physical experience, anchoring ourselves in the present moment through the most tangible and corporeal of connections.

The human body, a marvel of biological engineering, serves as a vessel for our very existence, providing us with an intimate and immediate window into the present moment. By cultivating a mindful awareness of our physical sensations, we can establish a direct line of communication with the present moment. Our senses can attune to the subtle vibrations, textures, and temperatures that make up our lived experience.

Consider, for a moment, the gentle brush of fabric against skin, the warmth of sunlight on one's face, and the delicate symphony of birdsong that graces our ears. In attending to these sensory experiences, we foster a more profound connection to the present moment, our awareness firmly embodied in the gift of physicality.

This embodied awareness invites us to inhabit our bodies with curiosity, compassion, and non-judgment to explore each sensation that arises within our corporeal form. As we engage in this practice, we may find ourselves becoming more attuned to the nuances of our physical experience and how that relates to our inner world as it fully merges with the now.

Mindfulness invites us to explore not only the realms of our thoughts and emotions but also the rich landscape of our physical experience. Embrace the practice of embodied awareness to allow the miraculous nature of your physical form to guide you further into the present moment.

⑤ Mindfulness in Action

Building upon all that we have covered so far, I must next impart upon you a revelation of sorts, a secret convenience that many who aspire to mindfulness are unaware is entirely at their disposal. This revelation, my dear friend, is the transformative power of mindfulness in action, a practice that weaves its way into even the most ordinary of tasks, transmuting them into opportunities for presence and awareness.

As we diligently cultivate our mindfulness practice, it offers us a chance to integrate its principles into every corner of our existence. When embraced wholeheartedly, the art of mindful living can imbue our days with a sense of wonder, appreciation, and presence, casting a luminescent glow upon the most mundane chores.

Imagine, for a moment, yourself engaged in the act of washing dishes, a task that has graced the lives of countless individuals since time immemorial. Through the lens of mindfulness, this seemingly trivial task can become a dance of sensation and awareness, our hands caressing the contours of each plate, our senses attuned to the gentle murmur of running water and the fragrant bouquet of soap.

Similarly, even the act of walking about the home or workspace can become a meditation in motion, each step a mindful exploration of the interplay between our bodies and the earth, the rhythmic cadence of our breath harmonizing with the alternating motion and stillness of life and form that surrounds us.

In embracing the art of mindful living, we allow ourselves to navigate the currents of time with easy tranquility. No matter how seemingly insignificant, each moment becomes an invitation to presence and awareness, a chance to deepen our connection to the eternal now.

Weave the threads of mindfulness into the fabric of your daily life to transform even the most ordinary tasks into opportunities for presence and growth. In doing so, you may discover that mindful living is not simply a practice but a way of being, a vibrant source of contentedness that colors every aspect of our human journey.

⑥ The Ripple Effects of Mindfulness

Before we move on, allow me to share with you a most delightful truth, one that extends beyond the confines of our individual experiences and reaches outward to touch the lives of those around us. This truth, you see, lies in the ripple effects of mindfulness, a practice whose influence extends far beyond the shores of our own inner landscape.

When we engage in mindfulness, we do more than simply anchor ourselves in the present moment; we also cast a soothing stone into the tranquil waters of our collective consciousness, creating gentle ripples that reverberate through the fabric of our shared existence.

As we develop our capacity for presence, compassion, and understanding, our relationships transform into vibrant expressions of connection and empathy. We learn to truly see one another, to recognize the radiant spark of humanity within every soul.

In turn, our communities increasingly become sanctuaries of harmony and cooperation, imbued with the timeless wisdom of mindfulness. We discover that our actions, no matter how small, can have a profound impact on the world around us and the trajectories of others, each choice and deed interlacing into our interconnected lives.

And ultimately, the ripple effects of mindfulness extend to the very fabric of our world, fostering a more compassionate, loving, and conscious existence for all. When we learn to live mindfully and embrace the eternal present with open hearts and minds, we create a space for healing, growth, and transformation—not only within ourselves but within the essence of our shared human journey.

So, let us venture forth into the world with the wisdom of mindfulness as our compass, nurturing the seeds of presence, compassion, and understanding within our hearts.

In doing so, we may find that the ripples we create extend far beyond our wildest dreams, transforming our relationships, our communities, and, ultimately, our world. As we develop our capacity for presence, compassion, and understanding, we foster a more harmonious and interconnected existence guided by the timeless wisdom of mindfulness.

XIX.

Balancing Acceptance and Change With the Scales of Serenity

In the multi-faceted flow of existence, we are continually called upon to manage the balance between acceptance and change, two seemingly contradictory forces that serve as the warp and weft of our ever-evolving reality.

As we journey along the path of personal growth and self-discovery, it is essential that we learn to integrate these dual aspects of life gracefully, allowing them to inform and enrich our experiences in equal measure. In this chapter, we shall explore the delicate interplay between acceptance and change, delving into the ways in which they can be artfully woven together to shape the life tapestry of our choosing.

 The Serenity Prayer

It is worth referring to an age-old adage, a jewel of wisdom that has graced the annals of history and enlightened countless souls on their journey through this beautiful life. The Serenity Prayer, as it is known, is attributed to the eminent theologian Reinhold Niebuhr and offers us a touchstone of guidance and discernment in our quest for balance and harmony.

Allow me to present this hallowed verse, a gleaming torchlight amidst the ever-changing seas of existence: "God, grant me the serenity to accept the things I cannot change, courage to change the things I can, and wisdom to know the difference."

In the spirit of this simple yet profound prayer, we find a roadmap for navigating the vicissitudes of life, a compass to guide us through the labyrinthine twists and turns of our shared human journey. To accept the things we cannot change, to recognize the immutable forces that shape the contours of our reality, is to embrace the essence of serenity, a state of tranquility and grace that anchors us amidst the storms of life.

And yet, we are also called upon to muster the courage to change the things we can, to take up the mantle of responsibility and forge a path towards a brighter, more expansive future. This dear reader, is the alchemy of transformation, the chrysalis from which our most authentic selves emerge, resplendent and free.

Finally, we are implored to cultivate the wisdom to know the difference between that which we can change and that which we cannot, a discernment that serves as a lodestar for our journey through the world. This subtle and impactful wisdom allows us to traverse the shifting tides of life with resilience and grace, guided by the unerring compass of the Serenity Prayer.

So, let us embrace the spirit of this age-old adage, allowing its wisdom to illuminate our path as we venture forth into the world, guided by the twin beacons of serenity and courage and the steadfast compass of discernment.

❷ The Paradox of Acceptance

There is a most intriguing paradox that lies at the very heart of our human experience. At first glance, acceptance may appear to be a passive, even defeatist state, one that requires us to resign ourselves to the whims of fate and circumstance. Yet, as we shall soon discover, the truth is far more layered and rich with nuance than it might initially seem.

Allow me to peel back the layers of this complex enigma, revealing the hidden depths that lie beneath the surface of our understanding. Contrary to popular belief, genuine acceptance is anything but passive; it is, in fact, a powerfully transformative force that enables us to seize the present moment in its entirety.

Picture, if you will, the supple branches of a willow tree, bending and swaying with the force of the wind, yet never breaking. This is the essence of true acceptance, a dynamic interplay between yielding and resilience, an interplay of surrender and strength that allows us to remain rooted in the fertile soil of the present moment.

As we learn to cultivate this state of acceptance, we discover that it is not, in fact, a retreat from the challenges of life but rather a deep and abiding engagement with the world as it truly is. From this vantage point, we can begin to discern the opportunities for growth, learning, and transformation that lie hidden within even the most testing of obstacles.

Within this enigmatic paradox of acceptance, we find the means to engage our most authentic, expansive, and fulfilling existence, discoverable thanks to the shining light of our own inner wisdom and the timeless truths that have illuminated the path of countless seekers who have gone before us.

③ The Catalyst of Change

Draw your attention to the ever-shifting landscape of our lives, where the winds of change blow both gently and fiercely, leaving no stone unturned, no tree unbent, and no horizon unaltered. Change, like acceptance, is an inherent aspect of existence, an ever-present force that shapes and reshapes our lives in countless and untold ways.

Yes, change can indeed be challenging, even painful, at times. Yet, as we shall soon uncover, it is also a vital catalyst for growth and transformation, inviting us to explore new possibilities and redefine the boundaries of our potential.

Picture, if you will, the mighty river that courses through the heart of a wild and untamed landscape, its waters carving a serpentine path through the earth, constantly shifting and flowing, yet always. This vision perfectly encapsulates the essence of change, a dynamic force that propels us onward, urging us to confront our fears and embrace the unknown.

As we navigate the rapids and currents of this ever-changing river of life, we may at times feel as though we are adrift, lost amid the restless tumult of the world. And yet, it is within these very moments of uncertainty and upheaval that we are presented with the most profound opportunities for growth, learning, and self-discovery.

So let us set sail upon these uncharted waters of change, courageously charting a course through the swirling eddies and crashing waves of life's ever-shifting currents.

In embracing the challenges and possibilities of change, we can begin to unlock the vast potential that lies dormant within every one of us, allowing us to forge a path that is uniquely our own and to create a life of boundless beauty.

 The Art of Discernment

Allow me to entreat your attention to a matter of great import, one that beckons us to traverse the intricate labyrinth of our existence. Within the hallowed halls of our inner sanctum, we are called upon to cultivate the art of discernment, a quietly mighty skill that permits us to better balance the tip of the scales between acceptance and change.

As we wend our way through the odysseys of our lives, we shall encounter moments when it is wise to surrender to the flow of life, to relinquish our resistance, and permit the currents of existence to carry us forward. Yet, there shall be occasions when it is necessary to take bold, purposeful action, to set our sails against the prevailing winds and chart our course through the vast ocean of life's possibilities.

Ah, discernment! This elusive and ephemeral skill, so difficult to define and yet so vital to our well-being, beckons us to refine our perceptions, to attune our senses to the subtle whispers of our intuition, and to attune our hearts to the wisdom of our innermost selves.

Picture in your mind's eye the master weaver, deftly intertwining the threads of acceptance and change into a rich and vibrant textile, a living testament to the beauty and complexity of our human experience. This, my dear reader, is the art of discernment in action, the ability to recognize when to steer into or ahead of the winds of change and when to find solace in the stillness of acceptance.

In honing our capacity for discernment, we are gifted with the opportunity to skillfully weave acceptance and change into the fabric of our lives, creating a more harmonious experience as we do. So let us embrace this art with open hearts and minds, for it is through the practice of discernment that we can begin to truly understand the intricate dance of life, finding grace and balance amid the ever-changing landscape of our shared human journey.

❺ <u>The Alchemy of Transformation</u>

I entreat you to accompany me on a quest of profound metamorphosis, a pilgrimage into the heartlands of the alchemy of transformation. As we plunge into the depths of our innermost selves, we are called upon to master the delicate interplay of acceptance and change to gracefully integrate these forces into the very fabric of our existence.

In this sense, the true alchemist carefully tends to the flames of transformation, transmuting the raw materials of experience, challenge, and insight into the shimmering gold of personal growth and self-discovery. This is the skill that we are invited to acquire, the sacred dance of transformation that beckons us to engage with the fullness of our being.

As we become more adept at the art of transformation, our lives are infused with the radiant light of our newfound wisdom and insight. We become like the mythic phoenix, rising from the ashes of our trials and tribulations, reborn into a more authentic, empowered, and radiant reality.

With each stage of this quest, we are gifted with the opportunity to forge a deeper connection with our truest selves, to embrace our experiences with open hearts and minds, and to share the light of our transformation with those who journey alongside us.

So, let us embark upon this pilgrimage with courage, curiosity, and compassion, for it is through the alchemy of transformation that we can genuinely begin to illuminate the path of our shared human journey, creating a more vibrant, expansive, and harmonious existence for ourselves and for all those who dwell within the embrace of our interconnected lives.

As we learn to gracefully integrate acceptance and change into our daily lives, we become adept at transformation, transmuting our experiences, challenges, and insights into the raw materials for personal growth and self-discovery.

As we go, let us remember that these seemingly opposing forces are, in fact, two sides of the same coin, essential aspects of the intricate dance of existence. By embracing both aspects equally, we can actively cultivate the art of discernment.

XX.

Nurturing Empathy and Compassion on the Path to Growth and Connection

Our capacity for self-awareness, growth, and transformation marks the flowering of the human spirit not only but also our ability to extend the tendrils of our hearts to encompass the experiences and emotions of others.

As we journey toward personal development, we must cultivate empathy and compassion, twin virtues that form the bedrock of our interconnectedness and serve as guiding lights in the unfolding narrative of our shared human experience.

In this chapter, we shall delve into the importance of empathy and compassion, exploring their transformative potential for both personal growth and the deepening of our connections with others.

① **The Nature of Empathy**

Let us venture together into the realm of empathy, that most essential of human faculties, which allows us to peer into the hearts and minds of our fellow travelers and to truly apprehend the subtleties of their inner worlds. Through this intimate exploration, we shall come to understand the intrinsic nature of empathy, the divine capacity that lies within each of us and which forms the foundation of our connections with one another.

As we stroll along this path, we encounter a multitude of souls, each with their unique experiences, thoughts, and emotions. As we do, empathy is the golden key that unlocks the door to these sacred inner sanctums, allowing us to step across the threshold and witness the world through the eyes of another.

To truly embody empathy, we must dissolve the boundaries that separate us, allow our hearts to be filled with the joys and sorrows of our fellow beings, and bear witness to the shared nature of the human experience. This, in turn, fosters a sense of unity, belonging, and shared humanity, a recognition that we are all, in essence, interconnected threads in the intricate web of existence.

As we cultivate this capacity for empathy, we are gifted with a profound insight into the very nature of our relationships, enabling us to forge more profound, more authentic connections with those alongside us on this journey of life. In so doing, we can begin to create a world that is guided by the principles of compassion, understanding, and mutual respect, a world in which each soul is honored, cherished, and nurtured.

Empathy, at its core, is the ability to perceive and understand the thoughts, feelings, and experiences of others, allowing us to step into their shoes and see the world from their perspective.

So, I entreat you to join me in embracing the transformative power of empathy, letting it guide and shape our interactions, and celebrating the beauty and wonder of our shared humanity, for it is through the nurturing of empathy that we can indeed come to know and understand the depths of our interconnectedness, and to weave harmony into our tapestries.

② The Gift of Compassion

I was hoping you could permit me to lead you through the lush gardens of compassion, that sublime and tender emotion that springs forth from the depths of our hearts and which so powerfully binds us together in a shared embrace of loving-kindness.

As we tread this path, hand in hand, we shall explore the myriad ways in which compassion can transform our lives, fostering a more expansive, generous, and authentic way of being in the world.

At the very heart of compassion lies the quivering of the heart, that sublime vibration that resonates through our very being when we bear witness to the suffering of another. This is the natural outpouring of empathy, the sweet nectar which flows from our ability to truly see and understand the pain and sorrow that resides within the hearts of our fellow beings.

As we open ourselves to this experience of compassion, we find that our hearts begin to swell with loving-kindness. This profound and unconditional love seeks to alleviate the suffering of others. This love, like unbroken sunlight, illuminates the darkest corners of our world, bathing our relationships, our communities, and our very selves in its radiant warmth.

In embracing the gift of compassion, we learn to see beyond the narrow confines of our own experience, to recognize the beauty and fragility of our shared humanity, and to extend our hands in acts of loving service guided by the boundless wisdom of our hearts.

To begin our compassionate awakening, not only hand in hand but also heart to heart, we must strive to create a world in which our participation becomes a chorus of love, a symphony of interconnectedness that reverberates through the very fabric of our existence. In so doing, we shall weave threads of compassion, forming a masterpiece of loving-kindness that will forever enshrine our shared humanity in the annals of time.

③ **The Empathic Bridge**

Let us examine the inner workings of empathy, the most exquisite human faculties that allow us to traverse the vast and varied landscape of human experience. As we journey together, let us delve into the depths of this extraordinary capacity for shared understanding and examine the ways in which it can foster a more inclusive, compassionate, and harmonious world, one in which we can all flourish and thrive.

Imagine people building bridges of understanding across the chasms of difference that so often divide us. These structures will be of such grace and beauty that they serve as a testament to the boundless potential of the human spirit.

My dear reader, these bridges are the essence of empathy, how we can connect with others across the most seemingly insurmountable barriers of culture, language, and experience.

In cultivating empathy, we create the possibility for genuine connection and shared understanding, building a foundation upon which we can foster a more compassionate and harmonious world. It is through the act of stepping into the shoes of another, of truly seeing the world through their eyes, that we can bridge the divides that have long separated us and recognize the beauty, the pain, and the fragile humanity that resides within us all.

As we nurture this capacity for shared understanding, we begin to weave mirroring connected tapestries, a masterpiece of unity stretching across the vast expanse of human experience. In so doing, we create a world where compassion, love, and understanding are guiding principles.

As we strive to build bridges of understanding that span the chasms of difference and unite us in a shared embrace of our common humanity, we forge a more inclusive and harmonious world, a world in which the very essence of empathy becomes the foundation upon which we build our shared future.

④ The Compassionate Heart

By embarking on a voyage into the depths of the compassionate heart, that most tender and vulnerable of human faculties enables us to bear witness to the suffering of others and respond with love, understanding, and a desire to ease their distress.

As we immerse ourselves in the intricacies of this most profound practice, we shall discover that the compassionate heart is not merely an instrument of solace for others but also a catalyst for our comfort, a means by which we may experience a more profound sense of love, connection, and belonging.

Imagine a world in which our hearts are so attuned to the suffering of others that we cannot help but respond with love and compassion, a world in which our capacity for empathy and understanding knows no bounds. In such a world, the boundaries that separate us reveal themselves as mirages, and we can recognize the shared humanity that resides within us all, irrespective of the external circumstances that might appear to divide us.

As we open our hearts to the suffering of others, we see that their pain is not separate from our own; that it is, in fact, a reflection of the same fragile, vulnerable, and beautiful humanity that exists within us all.

In this recognition, we find not only the impetus to ease their distress but also the potential for our transformation as our hearts expand to encompass the vastness of human experience wherever we encounter it.

Through compassion, we transform the lives of those around us and reshape our hearts, allowing us to experience a deeper and more profound sense of love, connection, and belonging. This is the genuine gift of a compassionate heart.

(5) Personal Growth Through Empathy and Compassion:

As you can see, on an adventure of self-discovery that leads us through the realms of empathy and compassion, those noblest virtues have the power to transform not only our relationships with others but also the essence of our being.

As we delve into the intricacies of these practices, we shall discover that empathy and compassion are more than mere tools for connection; they are, in fact, fuel for our own personal growth and development, challenging us to expand the boundaries of our self-awareness and become more open, understanding, and accepting of both ourselves and others.

Suppose we dare to dream that our capacity for empathy knows no bounds. In that case, we birth a world in which our hearts are so attuned to the thoughts, feelings, and experiences of others that we cannot help but respond with love, understanding, and a desire to alleviate their suffering.

In such a world, it would compel us to confront our own biases, assumptions, and judgments, for how could we truly empathize with another if the constraints of our own preconceptions shackled us?

In cultivating compassion, it invited us to open our hearts to the suffering of others, to recognize that their pain is not separate from our own, but rather, a reflection of the same fragile, vulnerable, and beautiful humanity that exists within us all.

As we embrace this practice, we not only deepen our connections with others but also foster our personal growth and development, for in opening our hearts to the suffering of others, we are also opening ourselves to the possibility of change and transformation.

As we nurture our capacity for empathy and compassion, we see these virtues are more than mere instruments of connection; they are an invitation to expand the boundaries of our self-awareness, challenge the assumptions and judgments that have shaped our lives, and embrace a more open, understanding, and accepting way of being in the world.

⑥ Casting Empathy and Compassion Into the Ripple

The exploration of the expansive and transformative power of empathy and compassion familiarizes us with virtues whose effects extend far beyond our personal relationships and might shape our society's very fabric.

As we together incorporate these noble practices, we discover they can deepen our connections with others and create a more just, equitable, and compassionate society in which all beings can flourish and thrive.

As we cultivate these virtues within ourselves, we begin to exert further influence over the ripples of change that extend far beyond our personal sphere.

Essentially, we are intentionally shaping that pebble dropped into a still pond, and in doing so, our acts of empathy and compassion send waves of kindness and understanding out into the world, touching the hearts and lives of those around us and inspiring them to carry these seeds of connection forward in their own lives.

These ripples of empathy and compassion can transform our personal relationships, our communities, and those beyond them. As we become more attuned to the experiences and emotions of others, we contribute to the creation of justice and equity and a society that elevates the needs and well-being of all with care and consideration.

In this world, empathy and compassion would nurture the emergence of a new paradigm of connection and shared humanity. The barriers of race, religion, gender, and social status would be transcended, giving rise to a more inclusive, diverse, and harmonious global community. We would witness the birth of a world in which all beings can flourish, united by the common thread of empathy and compassion that binds us all together.

> **So embrace the transformative power of empathy and compassion, and embark on this journey of connection and shared humanity.**

XXI.

Practical Empathic Strategies for Cultivating Emotional Intelligence

The capacity to perceive and understand the emotions of others, as well as to navigate the intricacies of our emotional landscape, is paramount in our journey toward personal growth and the forging of deep, meaningful connections.

In the service of this vision, empathy and emotional intelligence, like all skills, can be honed and developed through practice and conscious effort. In this chapter, we shall explore a range of practical strategies designed to cultivate empathy and emotional intelligence, empowering us to become more compassionate, understanding, and emotionally attuned individuals.

1. Active Listening

Active listening is an art that serves as the very foundation of empathy and lies at the heart of our shared human experience. Through this practice of genuinely hearing another person, we demonstrate our genuine interest in understanding their thoughts and feelings and, in doing so, allow ourselves to enter their worldly tapestries and share in their experiences.

Imagine, if you will, the nourishing and intricate transaction that occurs when two souls engage in active listening. Picture the delicate interplay of thoughts and emotions, the giving and receiving of understanding, and the shaping of a shared experience that solidifies human connection. This exchange, my dear reader, is one of profound intimacy, of vulnerability, and trust; indeed, empathy in action.

To develop the art of active listening, we must first learn to give our undivided attention to the speaker, focusing not only on the words they speak but also on the emotions and intentions that lie beneath the surface. In doing so, we must resist the urge to judge or interrupt and instead seek to understand their perspective with an open and compassionate heart.

One may liken this process to the act of cradling a delicate flower in one's hand, taking care not to crush its fragile petals or disturb its intricate beauty. Likewise, we must approach the thoughts and feelings of others with a similar gentleness and reverence, recognizing the inherent worth and dignity that lives within each and every soul.

As we hone our skills in active listening, we not only deepen our capacity for empathy and understanding but also create a fertile ground for the seeds of compassion to take root and grow. Moreover, in nurturing these virtues within ourselves, we foster a more authentic and connected way of being in the world, allowing us to cultivate relationships that are rich in love, trust, and understanding.

Taking part in active listening means embracing the art of truly hearing one another and the transformative power it holds. In doing so, we shall not only cultivate empathy and compassion within ourselves but also contribute to the creation of a more connected, harmonious, and compassionate journey for all.

 Mindful Awareness

Mindful awareness is an indispensable tool in the quest for emotional intelligence, and it is through this mindful attentiveness to our emotional states we can navigate the ebb and flow of our inner world with skill and self-care.

If you will, picture the myriad of emotions that make up the rich tapestry of human experience. Each thread is a unique shade and hue that combines to form the intricate patterns of our inner lives. Though often vague and transient, these emotions hold within them a wealth of wisdom and insight, waiting to be uncovered by those who dare to dive into their depths.

To cultivate mindful awareness of our emotions, we must first become attuned to the subtle nuances that permeate our emotional repertoire. This requires a level of presence and attentiveness akin to the delicate touch of a master painter, who constantly discovers and then handpicks each new color and applies it with precision and care.

One of the most effective ways to incorporate mindfulness into our daily routine is to set aside time for meditation or engage in activities that promote self-reflection and introspection.

Though uncomplicated, these practices have the potential to yield profound insights into the inner workings of our emotional lives, allowing us to develop a deeper understanding of ourselves and the world as we meet them.

As we become more adept at recognizing and responding to our emotions, we strengthen our emotional intelligence and foster a more compassionate and empathetic way of being in the world. In addition, through mindful awareness, we learn to see ourselves and others with greater clarity, allowing us to respond to life's events with greater stability.

Developing emotional intelligence requires cultivating a mindful awareness of our own emotional states. By practicing mindfulness, we can become more attuned to the subtle nuances of our emotions, allowing us to respond to them more skillfully and compassionately. In doing so, we shall not only enrich our lives but also contribute more broadly as we recognize the emotional tides that wash across the lives of others.

❸ Emotional Vocabulary

The intimate chambers of our emotional lexicon offer a veritable treasure trove of words and phrases that can illuminate the deepest recesses of our inner lives. In this expansive realm of language, we can give voice to our most profound feelings and, in turn, gain a richer understanding of ourselves and others.

As we embark on this linguistic sojourn, let us consider the vast array of emotions that constitute the human experience, each with its own distinct hue and character. From the subtlest shades of melancholy to the most vibrant tones of joy, the emotional spectrum is a kaleidoscope of nuance and complexity, waiting to be explored through the artful use of language.

To expand our emotional vocabulary, we must first consciously seek out new words and phrases that capture the essence of our emotions. We can return to the metaphor of that painter who continually refines their palette, and in mirroring that tendency, we too can broaden our emotional lexicon by immersing ourselves in literature, poetry, and the richness of human expression that surrounds us.

As we encounter unfamiliar words and phrases, let us not shy away from incorporating them into our daily conversations, for it is through practice that we enhance our emotional literacy. By giving voice to our feelings, we deepen our connections with others and create a more authentic and empathetic way of being in the world.

Expanding our emotional vocabulary enables us to better understand and express our feelings, as well as those of others. Make a conscious effort to learn new words and phrases to describe emotions, and practice using them in conversation to enhance your emotional literacy as we pursue this journey of linguistic discovery together.

 Perspective-Taking

The exploration of perspective-taking is a most essential and illuminating facet of empathy. In doing so, we shall plumb the depths of our imagination, a realm where the boundaries of self and others begin to blur, and the heart expands to encompass the myriad experiences of our fellow human beings.

To develop this adaptive and transformative skill, I invite you to engage in exercises that challenge your mind to adopt the viewpoint of another. Imagine stepping into a stranger's shoes, feeling the weight of their cares and concerns, and seeing the world through their eyes. Let this exercise serve as a portal to understanding as you traverse the unfamiliar landscapes of their lives.

Consider, too, the art of role-playing, a practice that invites you to assume the identity of another temporarily to explore their thoughts, feelings, and motivations. By immersing yourself in their world, you create a bridge of understanding that spans the chasm of difference, fostering a more profound sense of connection and compassion.

As you engage in these exercises, you may find your worldview expanding, your heart opening, and your capacity for empathy deepening. The practice of perspective-taking not only enhances our understanding of others but also enriches our own lives, for it is through the eyes of another that we can glimpse previously unseen facets of our shared humanity. Without a doubt, the cornerstone of empathy is the ability to see the world from another person's perspective.

❺ Nonverbal Communication

Let us next enter the domain of nonverbal communication, that unspoken medley of cues and signals that convey the subtleties of our emotions and intentions. As we enter the domain of nonverbal communication, I invite you to sharpen your senses and attune yourself to the nuances of human interaction.

We can reveal the richness of our connections by paying attention to these details.

It is said that a picture paints a thousand words, and so do the myriad expressions that flit across our countenance, the gentle sway of our bodies, and the cadence of our voices. To enhance your emotional intelligence, I urge you to become a keen observer of these nonverbal cues, for they are the silent song that underpins our interactions.

As you attune yourself to this language without words, I encourage you to practice the art of mirroring, a gentle act of empathy that involves subtly reflecting another person's body language and emotional state. When done with intention and sensitivity, this practice can foster a deeper sense of connection and understanding between individuals.

Envision the delicate arch of an eyebrow in response to a shared secret, the comforting touch of a hand on the shoulder in a moment of grief, or the warmth of a smile that ignites the embers of connection. When skillfully mirrored, these nonverbal cues can serve as a balm to the soul, a testament to the power of empathy and compassion.

A significant portion of our communication is conveyed through nonverbal cues, such as facial expressions, body language, and tone of voice. Embrace the subtle arts of nonverbal communication and mirroring, and in doing so, enhance your emotional intelligence as you forge deeper, more meaningful connections with fellow travelers on this wondrous journey we call life.

6. Cultivating Empathy Through Literature and Art

The historied chronicles of literature and art serve as hallowed sanctuaries of human expression that reveal the inner workings of the soul. As we explore them, let us open our hearts and minds to the myriad perspectives that lie within, for it is in the exploration of these diverse narratives that we can cultivate a new layer of empathy and emotional intelligence.

Picture yourself immersed in the pages of a novel, entering the world of its characters and experiencing their joys and sorrows, triumphs and tragedies.

As we throw ourselves into these stories, we bridge the gap between our own lives and those of others, forging connections that transcend time and space. Through these literary encounters, we also manifest a portal into the emotions and experiences of its creators, allowing us to bear witness to the depths of their humanity.

Gaze upon a painting, and imagine the artist's hand, guided by a wellspring of emotion, as they bring their vision to life on the canvas. Stand before a sculpture and contemplate the artist's intention as they transform raw material into an expression of their innermost thoughts and feelings.

By immersing ourselves in the worlds of literature and art, we engage in empathic manifestation, transmuting the insights and emotions we encounter into a deeper understanding of ourselves and others. As we navigate these chronicles, let us remember that each story, each brushstroke, each chisel mark, is a testament to the universality of the human experience, a reminder of our shared humanity.

⓻ Emotional Self-Regulation

In the grand theatre of life, emotions take center stage, their performance captivating and enthralling us in a dance of joy, sorrow, passion, and tranquility. Yet, as the curtain rises and falls on each act, we must learn to master the art of emotional self-regulation, an essential component of emotional intelligence that allows us to orchestrate our inner symphony with grace and finesse.

Place an imagined version of yourself in a moment of heightened emotion as the delicate balance of your inner world trembles on the edge of discord. It is in these moments that we must call upon our repertoire of self-regulation techniques, the conductor's baton that guides our emotional ensemble through the crescendos and diminuendos of life's richly representative soundscape.

Take, for instance, the simple yet potent act of deep breathing, a practice that can restore harmony to the cacophony of our emotional state. Inhale deeply, fill your lungs with the rejuvenating breath of life, and then exhale slowly, releasing the accumulated tension. With each breath, feel the gentle flow of your emotions as they surrender to the soothing rhythm of your respiration.

Or consider the art of progressive muscle relaxation, a method that invites us to explore the landscape of our physical form and the many tensions that often reside within. Begin at the crown of your head and journey downward, consciously releasing the clenched muscles and unspoken emotions that lie hidden beneath the surface. As you proceed, feel the weight of stress and disquiet melt away, revealing a serene and tranquil oasis.

Last, let us turn our gaze to the realm of visualization, a powerful technique that allows us to harness the boundless potential of our imagination. Close your eyes and envision a sanctuary of peace and calm, a haven where your emotions can find solace and reprieve. As you explore this inwardly created space, allow the healing balm of tranquility to envelop your heart and mind, restoring equilibrium to your emotional world.

Thus, let us take up the conductor's baton and skillfully guide our emotional orchestra through the symphony of life. By mastering the skill of emotional self-regulation and proactively regulating our emotions in healthy and adaptive ways, we not only enhance our emotional intelligence but also compose a more harmonious, expressive, and authentic score for our existence.

8. Seek Feedback and Growth Opportunities

As we journey through the maze of life, we are presented with countless opportunities to refine our empathy and emotional intelligence capacities. Like an exquisite sculpture hewn from the raw marble of experience, we become the masterpieces we are destined to be through the process of chipping away at our imperfections and polishing our rough edges.

In the atelier of personal growth, feedback serves as a most invaluable tool, a chisel that reveals the hidden contours of our character and guides our hand as we shape our emotional selves. Imagine the vulnerability of laying bare one's soul, inviting the discerning eye of another to observe the intricacies of our emotional tapestry, and offering their insights into the threads that weave our inner worlds.

To welcome such feedback is an act of courage, a testament to our commitment to growth and self-improvement. As we open ourselves to the words of others, be they praise or critique, we must cultivate a spirit of receptivity, a willingness to embrace the lessons that lie concealed within their observations. It is through integrating these insights that we may begin to understand the complexity of our emotional landscape and the myriad ways in which it intertwines with the lives of those around us.

Moreover, we must not shy away from the growth opportunities that life so generously bestows upon us. Each encounter, every exchange, presents a chance to delve deeper into the realm of empathy and emotional intelligence to expand our understanding of the human experience and our place within it. So embrace these moments with an open heart and an eager mind, for they are the crucible in which our emotional wisdom is forged.

Actively seeking feedback from others and embracing opportunities for personal growth are essential to developing empathy and emotional intelligence. Be open to constructive criticism, and consciously learn from your experiences and interactions with others. By embracing these practical strategies, we can nurture our empathy and emotional intelligence, fostering a greater capacity for understanding, connection, and emotional attunement.

XXII.

Setting Realistic Goals for Personal Growth and Self-Improvement

In the boundless expanse of human potential, the ability to set realistic goals guides us toward the shores of self-improvement and personal growth. Far from mere wishes cast upon the winds of chance, these carefully crafted intentions empower us to navigate the ever-changing seas of life with purpose and determination.

In this chapter, we shall explore the significance of setting achievable goals and the role of embracing change in our quest for personal fulfillment and self-actualization.

① The Anatomy of Achievable Goals

The journey of self-improvement is akin to a grand and intricate musical composition, a masterful construction of goals, aspirations, and dreams, each note resonating within the chambers of our hearts.

Yet, the beauty of this layered anthem lies not merely in the soaring crescendos and tender melodies but rather in the meticulous craftsmanship of its composition, the intricate structure that supports and sustains the harmony of our personal growth.

As we continue our journey of self-discovery and transformation, we must arm ourselves with the tools of precision and clarity, the instruments with which to sculpt our aspirations into the tangible milestones that will guide our path. Here, within the anatomy of achievable goals, we find the blueprint for success, the pedestal upon which we build the edifice of our dreams.

In crafting these goals, we must adhere to the principles of **s**pecificity, **m**easurability, **a**chievability, **r**elevance, and **t**ime-bound nature, the tenets that form the very foundation of the SMART methodology. Through applying these principles, we imbue our objectives with the clarity and direction necessary to navigate the labyrinthine pathways of personal growth.

The first stroke of the pen, the first note in the symphony, begins with specificity. By clearly defining our aspirations, we create a tangible vision of our desired outcome, a spotlight that reveals our path through the shadows of uncertainty. By asking ourselves the pertinent questions—the who, what, when, where, and why—we bring our goals into sharp focus, crystallizing our intentions into the framework of our journey.

Next, we must ensure that our goals are measurable, quantifiable milestones that allow us to track our progress and celebrate our achievements. By establishing concrete indicators of success, we create a roadmap for our journey, a means by which to gauge our growth and adjust our course as necessary.

As we traverse the landscape of self-improvement, we must also be mindful of the achievability of our goals. It is here that we find the delicate balance between aspiration and realism, the nexus where our dreams intersect with the boundaries of possibility.

By setting attainable objectives, we lay the groundwork for sustainable progress, fostering a sense of confidence and self-efficacy that will fuel our continued growth.

Relevance, too, plays a crucial role in the anatomy of achievable goals. By aligning our objectives with our values, passions, and long-term vision, we ensure that our efforts are invested in the pursuits that truly resonate with our hearts, cultivating a sense of purpose and motivation that will sustain us throughout our journey.

Finally, we must anchor our goals within the constraints of time, establishing periodic deadlines that provide structure and urgency to our endeavors. By delineating the temporal boundaries of our aspirations, we create a sense of momentum and drive, propelling ourselves forward in the pursuit of our dreams.

Thus, as we set forth on the path of self-improvement, let us embrace the anatomy of achievable goals, the blueprint that will guide our journey through the symphony of personal growth. With specificity, measurability, achievability, relevance, and time-bound nature as our compass, we shall navigate the labyrinthine pathways of our aspirations, crafting a masterpiece of harmony, success, and fulfillment.

To pave the path to self-improvement, one must use the building blocks of well-defined, realistic goals. By establishing objectives that are **s**pecific, **m**easurable, **a**chievable, **r**elevant, and **t**ime-bound (SMART), we create a blueprint for success that provides clarity and direction in our personal growth journey.

② The Power of Incremental Progress

In pursuit of self-improvement, we often find ourselves seduced by the grandiose visions of success and accomplishment, the triumphant conquests that punctuate the narrative of our personal growth.

And yet, as we peel back the layers of this narrative, we discover that the true beauty lies not in the bold strokes of achievement but in the delicate threads of incremental progress, the subtle hues and nuances that weave together to form the whole.

As we embark upon the journey of self-improvement, we must recognize the essential presence of the smaller steps of incremental progress. This gentle yet relentless force shapes the contours of our aspirations. To harness this power, we must first break down our larger, long-term goals into smaller, manageable steps, the stepping stones that will guide us across the vast chasm of our dreams.

Each step, however minute, carries within it a sense of accomplishment, should we choose to recognize it, a quiet triumph that feeds our motivation and propels us forward. In these moments of subtle victory, we find the momentum to continue our ascent, to climb ever higher toward the pinnacle of our potential.

But to truly appreciate the power of incremental progress, we must also cultivate a spirit of patience and perseverance, a steadfast commitment to the gradual, iterative process of growth. In this unwavering resolve, we find the strength to follow our journey's winding pathways and navigate the obstacles and challenges that will inevitably arise.

As we progress, let us not forget to celebrate these minor victories, to savor the sweet taste of accomplishment that accompanies each step. In doing so, we foster a sense of self-efficacy, a belief in our ability to conquer the seemingly insurmountable peaks that loom before us.

And as we weave together the threads of incremental progress, let us also remember the value of reflection, of pausing to survey the landscape of our growth and taking stock of the distance we have traveled. In these moments of introspection, we gain a deeper understanding of ourselves and a newfound appreciation for the intricate nature of life's inevitable momentum.

③ Embracing the Winds of Change

We often find ourselves adrift and rolling across the cresting waves of change, buffeted by the winds of fortune and fate, as we strive to navigate the uncharted waters of our aspirations. Yet, in these moments of vulnerability and uncertainty, we discover the true measure of our character, the resilience, and adaptability that define the contours of our personal growth.

As we ride out each storm, it is of paramount importance that we cultivate a mindset of flexibility and resilience. This mental alchemy transmutes the leaden weight of adversity into the golden wings of opportunity. In this melting pot of transformation, we fashion our destiny, constructing a thread of triumph from the gossamer fibers of change.

To embrace the winds of change, we must first learn to relinquish our attachment to the familiar, the comforting swaddles of our past. In this act of surrender, we find the strength to venture forth into the unknown.

As we journey through the tempest of change, let us cultivate a spirit of resilience, a steadfast resolve to persevere in adversity, for it is in this unwavering determination that we find the power to weather the storm, to endure the trials and tribulations that lie in wait upon the path of our pursuit.

And as we embrace the winds of change, let us not forget the importance of reflection, of pausing to savor the lessons gleaned from our experiences. In these moments of introspection, we gain a deeper understanding of ourselves and a newfound appreciation for the mutable nature of our existence.

Thus, as we navigate the ever-shifting landscape of life, let us be emboldened by the knowledge that only with courage can we manifest the masterpiece of our personal growth. Through adaptability and resilience, we shall conquer the tempest, rising triumphantly upon the wings of our growth to soar ever higher toward the boundless horizon.

 The Importance of Self-Reflection

With due diligence, the pursuit of self-improvement can guide our steps toward the shimmering summit of our aspirations.

But, first, one must not overlook the importance of self-reflection — a potential series of way stones along our path, providing the clarity and insight necessary to chart our course through the ever-changing landscape of personal growth.

Amidst the whirlwind of our daily lives, it is all too easy to become lost amidst the tangle of routine and distraction, losing sight of the overarching purpose that lies at the heart of our ambitions. In these moments of disorientation, we must seek a moment of quiet sanctuary and introspection, pausing in a hallowed space where we may delve into the inner recesses of our being and take stock of our progress thus far.

As we self-explore, we are called upon to scrutinize the countless facets of our experience with a discerning eye, sifting through the layers of our thoughts, emotions, and actions in search of the gems of wisdom that lie stowed within. By assessing our progress, identifying areas of growth, and recalibrating our goals accordingly, we ensure that our ambitions remain aligned with our evolving needs and desires.

In this state of self-reflection, we also confront our own shortcomings and the shadows that lurk within the uncharted depths of our psyche. Through this process of unearthing and acknowledging our limitations, we turn a handle on the door to self-improvement, casting aside the shackles of stagnation and complacency that hinder our ascent toward the pinnacle of our potential.

As we embrace the practice of regular self-reflection, we cultivate a mindset of continuous learning and adaptation, instilling within ourselves the resilience and agility necessary to navigate the ever-shifting currents of our lives. This ceaseless cycle of introspection and recalibration serves as the engine that drives our journey toward self-mastery, propelling us ever onward in pursuit of the elusive next peak of personal growth.

Thus, let us heed the call to self-reflection, embracing the profound insights and revelations that arise from this intimate communion with our innermost selves. Through this sacred act of introspection, we shall chart the course to a brighter, more enlightened future, setting our sights upon the distant mountaintops of self-improvement and embarking upon the grand odyssey of our lives with renewed vigor and purpose.

Regular self-reflection serves as a crucial checkpoint on our journey toward self-improvement. By assessing our progress, identifying areas of growth, and recalibrating our goals accordingly, we ensure that our ambitions remain aligned with our developing needs and desires.

⑤ Balancing Ambition and Acceptance

As we step into each day's unwavering light, the ever-oscillating pendulum of ambition and acceptance, each resonant swing shaping the trajectory of our personal evolution, inevitably beset us.

Between these swings, we must learn to strike a harmonious balance. This act requires a keen eye for the subtleties of our desires and a profound understanding of the intricate interplay between aspiration and contentment.

As we traverse the winding pathways of our existence, the relentless pursuit of our ambitions often drives us, the shimmering gloss of achievement beckoning us forward with its siren song of progress and self-improvement. Yet, in our relentless quest for growth, it is all too easy to become entangled in the intoxicating allure of attainment, losing sight of the present moment and the exquisite beauty of our current circumstances.

Vitally, we must learn to temper our desires with the soothing balm of acceptance, acknowledging the inherent worth of our current situation and embracing the invaluable lessons it offers. Within the embrace of acceptance, we find the seeds of wisdom that nourish our growth, providing the fertile soil in which our aspirations may take root and flourish.

To cultivate this delicate equilibrium, we must first learn to recognize the discreet signals of our hearts, attuning ourselves to the whispers of our innermost longing and the unspoken yearnings hidden beneath the clamor of daily life.

Through this process of introspection, we may discern where ambition may masquerade before a truer ally of acceptance within our psyche, adjusting our steps to align with the ever-shifting rhythms of our souls.

There is much to be said for holding space for both our aspirations and our present circumstances, honoring the unique potential and wisdom that lives within each. In this delicate act of balancing ambition and acceptance, we find not only the key to our own growth but also the gateway to a more profound and authentic connection with ourselves and the world around us.

Thus, let us cultivate this harmonious equilibrium, traversing the intricate tightrope of ambition and acceptance with grace and poise to better bask in the luminosity of self-improvement and self-discovery.

The equilibrium between ambition and acceptance is the fulcrum upon which our personal growth hinges. While it is essential to strive for self-improvement, we must also cultivate the ability to accept and embrace our present circumstances, recognizing the inherent value and lessons they hold.

⑥ The Role of Accountability

Accountability serves as the steadfast metronome that guides our progress toward the lofty summits of self-improvement. As we assess and quantify our aspirations, it is the unwavering commitment to our goals and the steadfast acknowledgment of our actions that provide the rudder, steering us through the intermittent mists of uncertainty and doubt.

Yet, as solitary creatures adrift in the vast ocean of our own desires, we often find ourselves in need of a guide, a gentle hand to steady our course and ensure that our course remains steadfastly aligned with the beacon of our aspirations. It is in these moments of vulnerability that we turn to those whom we hold dear, seeking solace and support within the loving embrace of our trusted confidants.

By enlisting the aid of friends, family, or mentors, we forge a powerful alliance that serves not only as a bulwark against the creeping tendrils of self-doubt and fear but also as a potent stimulant for our growth and development. Accountability always accompanies such a gift, as the shared camaraderie of our trusted allies facilitates the fortitude to view ourselves as responsible for our actions and progress.

In this sacred space of accountability, we are called to bear witness to our own growth, to confront the innermost recesses of our hearts, and lay bare the truths that reside therein.

For it is only in the self-examination and honest reflection within the mirror held by our confidants that we may truly embrace the mantle of accountability, reinforcing an unwavering commitment to our goals and aspirations that is tempered by the steadfast support of our loved ones.

Thus, let us stand tall in the face of adversity, holding ourselves accountable for our actions and progress as a vital component of successful goal-setting. By enlisting the support of trusted friends, family, or mentors, we create a network of encouragement and accountability that bolsters our determination and commitment.

⑦ The Art of Perseverance

Perseverance reigns supreme as the indomitable force that propels us ever forward, surmounting the formidable peaks of adversity that loom large on the horizon. As we traverse the undulating terrain of our own personal growth, this unwavering resolve fuels our progress, propelling a trajectory that leads upward to the hallowed heights of self-actualization.

Yet, as we meander through the swaying limbs of our ambitions, the specters of setback and failure all too often meet us, their gnarled talons threatening to capture us in the lowland shadows of despondency and despair.

In these moments of darkness, when the flame of hope flickers precariously, we must call upon the inner reserves of resilience and grit that lie dormant within the depths of our souls.

For it is within the heat of perseverance that the true measure of our character is forged as we emerge from the ashes of defeat, strengthened by the fires of adversity. To nurture this indomitable spirit, we must cultivate a steadfast resolve that remains unshaken by the vicissitudes of fortune, refusing to yield in the face of obstacles or to the diversions of low-hanging branches.

As we embark upon this journey, we must arm ourselves with the twin swords of patience and tenacity, wielding them with unerring precision as we navigate the forest of our uncertainty and self-doubt. By honing our capacity for perseverance, we forge an unbreakable shield that protects us from the slings and arrows of misfortune, empowering us to overcome even the most daunting of challenges.

Therefore, let us embrace the art of perseverance with open hearts and open minds, drawing strength from the wellspring of resilience that resides within each of us, for it is only through the dogged pursuit of our goals and aspirations, undeterred by the looming specter of adversity, that we may ascend to the gilded pantheon of self-improvement, triumphant and resolute in our quest for personal growth.

In the face of setbacks and obstacles, the ability to persevere and maintain focus on our goals is the hallmark of personal growth. By developing resilience and grit, we can continue to move forward, undeterred by the challenges that arise on our journey toward self-improvement.

⑧ Celebrating Milestones and Successes

Embroidered with the myriad threads of ambition, adversity, and triumph, the moments of success, those shimmering jewels of achievement that sparkle most brilliantly against the backdrop of our adventure. As we embark upon this sometimes arduous trial of self-improvement, it is essential that we pause to celebrate the milestones we attain, those precious markers that tell us we are traveling in the direction intended.

In our accomplishments, we find the sustenance that nourishes our motivation and commitment, a veritable feast of inspiration that propels us ever onward in our quest for personal growth. In these moments of jubilation, as we bask in the warm glow of victory, we are reminded of the inestimable value of our efforts, fueling our fervor to press on toward greater heights.

Yet, it is not solely the grand achievements that warrant celebration. Still, the modest triumphs are those seemingly inconsequential victories that, when viewed in isolation, may appear insignificant but, in truth, form the buttresses that sure up our larger aspirations. These humble milestones serve as the props of progress, the incremental steps that, when taken in concert, pave the way for the realization of our most daring ambitions.

Let us, therefore, raise our voices in a jubilant chorus, extolling the virtues of our accomplishments, be they grand or humble, as we navigate the winding path of self-improvement. For it is in the celebration of these milestones that we find the nourishment that sustains us, the lifeblood of motivation that courses through our veins, invigorating and revitalizing our spirits as we forge onward in our relentless pursuit of personal growth.

By savoring these moments of triumph, we fuel our desire to continue on the path of self-improvement and actualization. So, as you celebrate your successes, both large and small, may you be filled with the unquenchable fire of ambition, the burning desire to scale the heights of self-improvement and actualization, buoyed by the knowledge that, with each milestone you celebrate, you draw ever closer to the summit of your choosing.

XXIII.
Practical Steps for Turning Long-Term Goals Into Manageable Tasks

The pursuit of long-term goals is akin to the intentional creation of our grand life tapestries, wherein each thread is woven meticulously to form a coherent and magnificent pattern. To successfully integrate the threads of personal growth and self-improvement, one must master the art of goal deconstruction—breaking down ambitious objectives into a series of manageable tasks. This chapter will investigate the practical steps necessary to transform lofty aspirations into tangible achievements.

① The Beauty of Specificity

As we navigate the vast and unmapped oceans of personal growth, the beauty of specificity serves as our sextant, the guiding indicator of clarity that measures our course and steers us true.

For in the realm of ambition, there is no navigational tool more steadfast nor more reliable than a well-defined, specific goal—a radiant vision that burns with the intensity of a thousand suns, casting a forward clarion light and beckoning us onward with its irresistible allure.

In the mosaic of our aspirations, the specificity of our long-term goals lends structure and coherence to the myriad tiles that comprise the tableau of our dreams. These goals, sharp and vivid in their precision, form the scaffolding upon which our ambitions are built, providing the support and stability necessary to scale the dizzying heights of self-actualization.

To distill the essence of our desires, we must begin by refining the ore of our ambitions, chiseling away the extraneous layers of vagueness and uncertainty until we are left with a pure, crystalline objective — a goal as specific and well-defined as the facets of a diamond, each angle, and plane expertly crafted to reflect the light of our dreams.

With this polished gem of clarity in hand, we are empowered to forge a path toward personal growth guided by the unwavering light of our long-term goal. This beacon of specificity, its luminescence undimmed by the mists of doubt and confusion, serves as our North Star, providing a sense of direction and purpose for the tasks that lie ahead.

So, as you embark upon this grand adventure of self-improvement, may you be fortified by the beauty of specificity, and may the radiant light of your well-defined goals serve as your guiding star, illuminating the path towards personal growth and leading you ever onward towards the fulfillment of your dreams.

Begin by clarifying the long-term goal, ensuring that it is specific and well-defined. A clear vision serves as the guiding star, illuminating the path toward personal growth and providing a sense of direction for the tasks that lie ahead.

❷ The Power of Reverse Engineering

In the quest for personal growth and the achievement of ambition, a potent and often underappreciated force holds the power to propel us toward our most audacious dreams—the art of reverse engineering.

Like a master clockmaker disassembling the intricate mechanisms of a timepiece, we, too, can deconstruct our ultimate objectives, revealing the hidden milestones and intermediary goals that form the component parts of our aspirations.

To harness the phenomenal power of reverse engineering, we must first cast our gaze upon a distant goalpost, allowing our eyes to alight upon the glittering prize of our ultimate objective. This temple of promise, gleaming with the possibility of success and accomplishment, serves as our starting point — the apex from which we shall descend, tracing the contours of our ambition in reverse.

With the pinnacle of our dreams firmly in mind, we begin the delicate process of unwinding the threads of our aspirations, teasing apart the intricate web of milestones and intermediary objectives that must be conquered along the way.

This meticulous dissection, undertaken with the precision of a surgeon's scalpel, lays bare the skeletal framework of our goal, enabling us to construct a detailed roadmap that charts our course toward the desired outcome.

As we delve deeper into the cave systems of our ambition, the power of reverse engineering becomes increasingly evident. The once-daunting monolith of our ultimate objective, now fragmented into its constituent elements, reveals itself as a series of manageable tasks and challenges, each a stepping stone that draws us inexorably closer to our goal.

By working backward from the summit of our dreams, we can more effectively navigate the treacherous terrain of personal growth, the precipices and pitfalls that stand between us and our desired destination.

With the power of reverse engineering at our disposal, we may chart a course toward success and accomplishment, fortified by the knowledge that each milestone identified and conquered brings us one step closer to the glorious realization of our ultimate objective.

As you venture forth into the realm of your aspirations, by deconstructing your dreams, may you wield the power of reverse engineering with deft skill and unwavering conviction, transforming the impossible into the attainable and the unattainable into the inevitable.

❸ The Art of Task Decomposition

We often encounter a formidable step on our journey—the seemingly insurmountable milestone. These titanic edifices of ambition, standing sentinel between us and our ultimate objectives, may appear daunting and impenetrable, their sheer magnitude enough to quell even the most ardent of spirits.

Fear not, dear reader, for there exists an artful technique to dismantle these behemoths and render them conquerable. We must simply further dismantle the obstacles in our way through the art of task decomposition.

Task decomposition, akin to creating recipes that allow us to recreate our most prized delights, is the process by which we dissect our milestones and intermediary objectives into smaller, even more, actionable tasks.

By breaking down the colossal goal into its constituent parts, we create a recipe for manageable and achievable progress, transforming the herculean task into a series of ingredients and instructions. One can implement these instructions one at a time.

To engage in this deconstruction, we must first focus on our milestone, scrutinizing it's every facet and nuance. Then, we inspect our milestone with the precision of a jeweler examining a precious gemstone and identify the cracks and fissures that form the weak points of our aim, the seams along which our goal may be cleaved and subdivided.

With these fault lines revealed, we set about the task of dissection, methodically separating our milestone into its component elements. Each of these smaller tasks, now liberated from the gargantuan mass of the original objective, serves as a rung on the ladder leading to our ultimate goal — a series of manageable challenges that, when surmounted, coalesce to form the grand tapestry of our ambition.

As we delve into the heart of our milestone, chipping away at its imposing facade with each successive task, the art of decomposition becomes our most steadfast ally. By reducing the formidable to the achievable and the monumental to the attainable, we unlock the door to progress and growth, emboldening ourselves to scale the once-daunting heights of our aspirations.

By dissecting the larger goal into its constituent parts, one creates a roadmap for manageable and achievable progress. With this formidable weapon in your arsenal, no milestone is too significant, and no obstacle is impossible — the world, and all its boundless possibilities, await.

 Prioritizing and Sequencing

We find ourselves confronted with a veritable panoply of tasks, each vying for our attention like a crowd's clamoring voices. Yet, amidst all these tasks clamoring for our attention, how can we distinguish which ones are urgent and which ones can wait?

The answer lies in the delicate mastery of prioritization and sequencing — a strategic approach to ordering our tasks based on urgency, importance, and feasibility, thus ensuring that our efforts are allocated efficiently and effectively.

Envision once more an artist's palette, each hue representing a distinct task that awaits attention. To create the masterpiece that is our ultimate objective, we must first determine the sequence in which these colors must be applied, carefully considering the interplay of hues and the balance of light and shade. It is through this meticulous arrangement that our priorities emerge, and our efforts coalesce into harmonious progress.

To successfully implement prioritization, we must first assess the urgency of our tasks. Those which carry the weight of deadlines or impending consequences should be placed at the forefront of our agenda. With the ticking clock as our constant companion, we attend to these time-sensitive matters with the utmost diligence, lest we fall victim to the relentless march of time.

Next, we turn our attention to the importance of each task, evaluating their significance in relation to our overarching goals. Like an auctioneer appraising the value of precious artifacts, we weigh the merits of each undertaking, prioritizing those that hold the greatest potential for growth and progress. By focusing our energies on these pivotal tasks, we ensure that our efforts are channeled toward the most critical aspects of our ambition.

Finally, we must consider the feasibility of our tasks, cognizant of the resources at our disposal and the constraints that bind us. With the pragmatism of a seasoned strategist, we sequence our tasks in a manner that maximizes our potential for success, allocating our efforts in accordance with the ebb and flow of circumstance and opportunity.

In the end, it is through the artful orchestration of prioritization and sequencing that we are able to navigate the terrain of our obligations. By taming the unruly chaos of competing tasks, we forge a path toward our goals, each carefully considered step propelling us ever closer to realizing our most cherished hopes.

So, begin the practice of determining the order in which your own tasks must be completed, prioritizing them based on urgency, importance, and feasibility. This strategic approach will ensure that your efforts are allocated in the most efficient, effective, and gloriously liberating manner possible.

⑤ Establishing Timeframes

We are often confronted with the passing of days and weeks as our goals grow no closer, casting their inexorably passing shadow across our endeavors.

As we continue to cast a gaze toward our goals, we find ourselves grappling in the perpetual tug of war between aspiration and the finite nature of time. Within this temporal struggle, the importance of establishing timeframes emerges, providing both structure and impetus to our most ardent pursuits.

The art of establishing timeframes requires a discerning eye and an intimate understanding of the tasks that lay before us. We must first assess the complexity of each undertaking, mindful of the intricate interplay of variables that may conspire to challenge our progress.

Like a fine watchmaker, we must calibrate our expectations in accordance with the intricacies of each task, ensuring that our deadlines are grounded in the realm of possibility.

In tandem with evaluating complexity, we must also consider any potential obstacles or dependencies that may impede our progress. With the foresight of a seasoned navigator, we anticipate the ebbs and flows of circumstance, charting a course that accounts for the unpredictable turbulence of life.

Having meticulously assessed the nature of our tasks, we are then poised to assign realistic timeframes for their completion. These temporal guideposts serve to instill a sense of urgency, compelling us to seize the fleeting moments that comprise our days.

It is within these carefully delineated timeframes that we find the impetus to propel ourselves toward our ultimate goal, the alluring call of deadlines urging us ever forward.

And so we embark, guided by the cadence of deadlines and the rhythm of accountability. As we waltz through the many hallways of our aspirations, establishing timeframes directs our energies and ensures that each movement is harnessed to pursue our most cherished dreams.

⑥ Cultivating Consistency

The threads of our aspirations intertwine, weaving an intricate narrative of dreams and desires. Yet, as we knowingly follow the meandering and milestone pathways that lead toward our long-term goals, we are confronted with a simple yet profound truth: consistency is the lifeblood of progress.

Like our diligent artist friend who labors over each brushstroke, or the devoted musician who tirelessly refines their technique, it is through consistency that we breathe life into the ambitions that live deep within our hearts.

Envision, if you please, the splendid image of a tree, its roots firmly entrenched within the earth, its branches stretching towards the heavens above. As the tree grows, its limbs reach ever skyward, nourished by the steady rhythm of nature's cycles. In much the same way, we, too, must cultivate consistency, nurturing the roots of our aspirations with the sustenance of routine and structure.

To develop a consistent routine, we must first cast our gaze upon the vast expanse of our days, surveying the landscape of our schedules with a discerning eye.

Then, with the precision of a master cartographer, we delineate the contours of our time, carving out sacred and mindful spaces within which our goals may flourish.

These sanctuaries, set aside for the sole purpose of nurturing our dreams, become the fertile soil from which the seeds of our aspirations take root and blossom.

As we forge our daily schedule, we must be cognizant of the charge and depletion of our energies, aligning our most critical tasks with the moments in which we are most attuned to the demands of our goals. By harnessing the natural rhythms of our lives, we create a synergy that amplifies our productivity and moves us toward our objectives.

In crafting our routine, we must also be vigilant in the face of temptation, guarding against the siren call of procrastination and distraction. Yet, like a steadfast sentinel, we maintain our resolve, resolute in our dedication to the sacred spaces of our schedule. It is within the embrace of consistency that we find the momentum to propel our dreams skyward, each incremental step an affirmation of our unwavering commitment.

So, as we continue in the merry chase towards our long-term goals, let us cultivate consistency with the tenderness of a loving caregiver, nurturing the delicate potential of our aspirations with the life-giving sustenance of routine and structure. In leveraging the power of consistency to breed progress, we set the stage for our dreams' steady and sustainable growth and the gradual unfolding of our desires.

7 Embracing Flexibility

The choreography of our days is often a delicate balance between the ebb and flow of our aspirations and the ever-shifting landscape of our circumstances. As we pirouette through our existence, we are confronted with an undeniable truth: the path to self-improvement is not a rigid, immutable course but rather a fluid, malleable voyage shaped by the capricious whims of fate and the winds of change.

As we attempt to find a current rhythm, we must embrace the art of flexibility, cultivating an adaptive spirit that enables us to navigate changes in tempo with grace and aplomb. Like the supple branches of our friend the willow tree, we bend but do not break, our resilience a testament to our capacity for growth and transformation.

To embody this spirit of flexibility, we must first acknowledge the inherent impermanence of our plans and priorities, recognizing that the roadmap we have charted may require revision and recalibration as we traverse the terrain of our lives.

With the keen eye of a bold explorer, we must be prepared to retrace our steps, reassessing the course we have laid out and adapting our trajectory as the need arises.

This willingness to embrace change, to pivot and adapt in the face of adversity, is the hallmark of actual personal growth. For it is not in the rigid, unyielding adherence to our plans that we find our greatest potential, but rather in the supple, fluid dance of adaptation and perseverance that we discover the depths of our strength and resilience.

As we journey onwards, let us take solace in knowing that the winds of change, though they may buffet us and challenge our resolve, ultimately propel us forward, the gales of adversity shaping us into more formidable versions of ourselves. With each gust, we learn to bend and sway, our flexibility a testament to our growth, our adaptability, the lifeblood of our evolution.

So, as we stride into the unknown, let us embrace the beauty of flexibility, recognizing the transient nature of our plans and priorities and cultivating the capacity for adaptation and change within ourselves. In doing so, we set the stage for a journey of self-improvement that is as fluid and dynamic as the ever-shifting landscape of our lives.

8 Monitoring Progress

In the hallowed chambers of our inner sanctum, the mirrored reflections of our aspirations confront us either as specters of our dreams and desires or allies who may reach through the translucent surface and aid our journey.

As we gaze into this looking glass of the soul, we are granted a rare opportunity for introspection and self-assessment, a chance to examine the quality of this alignment by measuring our progress toward our ambitions.

In this sanctified space, we must embrace the ritual of monitoring progress, the quiet, contemplative act of bearing witness to the fruits of our labor and the incremental advances we have made along the twisting path of personal growth. With the watchful eye of a seasoned critic, we review and evaluate the tasks we have undertaken, the milestones we have crossed, and the obstacles we have surmounted in our quest for self-improvement.

This self-assessment process is unlike the art of navigation, with the celestial bodies of our accomplishments and shortcomings serving as guiding stars in the firmament of our journey. By charting our progress, we are able to identify areas of growth and opportunities for course correction, ensuring that our voyage remains aligned with the compass of our truest desires.

As we commit to this introspective practice, we must be prepared to confront the stark realities of our successes and failures, embracing the wisdom that lies within the unvarnished truth of our experiences. In doing so, we replace specters with allies, refining and recalibrating our roadmap and honing our trajectory with the precision of one use to standing at the helm.

In this intimate communion with the self, we bear witness to the alchemy of our evolution, the slow, inexorable transformation that unfurls within our souls. As we monitor our progress, we become the architects of our destiny, the custodians of our dreams, and the guardians of our personal growth.

Thus, let us pledge ourselves to the sacred art of self-assessment, the ritual of monitoring progress, a vital touchstone on the journey towards self-improvement. In this practice, we find the clarity and direction we seek.

> **Through the artful deconstruction of long-term goals into manageable tasks, one can transform the impossible into the eminently achievable. By approaching personal growth and self-improvement with a strategic mindset and a dedication to progress, the grand plan of one's ambitions becomes a reality woven with the threads of determination, persistence, and unwavering focus.**

XXIV.

Embracing Change in the Face of Life's Uncertainties

In the roadways of existence, the traffic of life flies past us in a dazzling display of movement and rhythm dictated by the ever-changing tempo of the human experience.

As we steer through that unpredictable flow on our journey, we are faced with the undeniable truth that change is the only constant. Yet, we find the keys to personal growth and self-improvement in the graceful acceptance and adaptation to this ever-shifting landscape.

① The Ephemeral Nature of Existence

In the quiet recesses of our hearts, we find ourselves confronted by the enigmatic presence of impermanence, the ephemeral nature of existence casting its veil across the details of our lives.

As we witness this dependable changeability, we are privy to the subtle shifts that define the landscape of our relationships, the waxing, and waning of affection, the blossoming and withering of love.

These fleeting moments, like the delicate petals of a cherry blossom, capture the essence of life's transience, the evanescent beauty that emerges and vanishes in the blink of an eye.

Beyond the confines of our existence, we witness the sweeping transformations wrought by the hurried flow of time, the tide of global events that shape the course of history and reshape the contours of the world. In this incredible story of change, we find ourselves but transient players, the notes of our lives resonating briefly before fading into the annals of eternity.

Faced with this ever-shifting panorama, we must embrace the wisdom that lies within the heart of impermanence, the understanding that life is a kaleidoscopic array of hues, an endless cascade of beginnings and endings, of creation and dissolution.

Through this acceptance, we awaken to the profound beauty of existence, the fleeting moments of joy and sorrow that illuminate the human experience like the flickering stars in the sky of our lives.

In this recognition, we find solace in the knowledge that change is the essence of life, the constant thread that weaves the fabric of our existence. In the gentle embrace of impermanence, we discover the freedom to live fully and authentically, savor each moment's transient beauty, and cherish the precious tapestry of our lives, with all its intricate and unexpected patterns.

Thus, let us celebrate the ephemeral nature of existence, the fleeting dance of change that defines the human experience. From the subtle shifts in our relationships to the sweeping transformations wrought by global events, change is an omnipresent force that defines the human experience.

In this recognition, we find the key to unearthing the hidden treasures of life, the wisdom to embrace the impermanent beauty that lies at the heart of our being, and the courage to live with authenticity, grace, and wonder.

(2) The Illusion of Control

Within the presence of our innermost thoughts, we encounter the disquieting realization that the threads of control, which we so desperately seek to grasp, often elude our most sincere efforts. In this life, we are but bit players, our influence extending only so far as the confines of our existence and the boundaries of our sphere of influence.

It is a humbling recognition, this admission that the world beyond our grasp is vast and intricate, formed by untold circumstance and fate, over which our control is but a fleeting illusion.

In the quietude of introspection, we find ourselves confronted by the sobering truth that the external forces that shape our lives are often beyond our ken, the capricious winds of fortune blowing hither and thither with nary a thought for the desires that burn within our hearts. The futile desire to control that beyond our reach is a lure that leads only into the treacherous waters of disillusionment and despair.

Yet faced with this disconcerting reality, we find the raft of understanding that our true strength lies not in the dominion we wield over the external world but in the fortitude and resilience that we cultivate within our hearts.

By acknowledging the limitations of our control, we relinquish the fruitless pursuit of mastery over that which is not ours to command, and in doing so, we open ourselves to the empowering potential of adaptability and resilience.

In this newfound liberation, we discover the freedom to chart our course, to navigate the turbulence of life with confidence and dexterity, our sails filled with the invigorating winds of adaptability and determination. We find that our true power lies not in the control we wield over the world but in the mastery we exercise over our own thoughts, emotions, and actions, the sovereignty we claim over the realm of our reactive natures.

So, let us embrace the illusion of control for what it truly is: a fleeting hallucination that dissipates like the morning mist beneath the sun's warm rays.

In its place, let us cultivate the resilience and adaptability that empowers us to weather the storms of life and emerge fruitful, our spirits undaunted by the whims of fate. In relinquishing control, we find the true essence of our strength, the indomitable spirit that lies at the very core of our being.

③ The Virtue of Adaptability

As we draw upon our minds in order to meet the waking world, we often find ourselves ensconced within walls of our own making, the familiar contours of our convictions and beliefs shaping the perimeters of our thoughts.

This provides the comfort of familiarity, yet within these very walls, we may discover the truth of our own confinement, the rigidity of our thinking, and the inflexibility of our beliefs stifling the growth and transformation that lie at the heart of the human experience.

To navigate beyond such self-constructed edifices, we must cultivate a mindset of flexibility and open-mindedness, a mental suppleness that allows us to move through the portals of circumstance and change. This dexterity of thought is the foundation upon which we can build our capacity for adaptation and resilience and fortify our ability to explore ever-expanding inner territories.

When we accept life's messages, we find that our most cherished beliefs and convictions are often tested and challenged, the immutable truths we once held dear melting away beneath the scorching heat of experience and wisdom.

In these moments of trial, flexibility reveals its true worth, allowing us to reshape and reform our thoughts and beliefs and elevate our very selves.

By embracing a mindset of flexibility and open-mindedness, we free ourselves from the manacles of our rigidity, and our hearts and minds are open to the world's boundless possibilities. We find that the limits of our thinking no longer constrain our capacity for growth and transformation, the vistas of our potential expanding beyond the horizons of our previous imaginings.

And so, let our spirits be buoyed by virtue of flexibility and the promise of growth and transformation that it holds, for it is in the openness to change, in the willingness to adapt and evolve, that we find the accurate measure of our resilience. This unyielding strength lies at the very core of our being.

 The Art of Reinvention

Within each of our personal histories, some chapters remain more indelibly etched upon the parchment of our souls than others, moments of metamorphosis that have forever altered the course of our lives. These transformative experiences beckon us to the threshold of reinvention, inviting us to evoke an inner reiteration, a reformulation that raises us above the vantage point of our former selves.

The art of reinvention is a refined craft, a finespun transformation that requires the courage to face the unknown and the humility to acknowledge the imperfections and limitations of our current selves. It is a journey of self-discovery and self-realization, a voyage into the yet unseen aspects of our souls in search of the hidden capabilities and understanding that wait beneath the surface of our consciousness.

As we progress through life, we must learn to view both internal and external change not as a harbinger of chaos and upheaval but as an opportunity to reimagine and redefine ourselves. By embracing the process of reinvention, we create the space for personal growth and the emergence of a more authentic and evolved self, a self that is better equipped to navigate the challenges and uncertainties that lie ahead.

With each iteration of our being, we shed the layers of our past selves like a snake sloughing off its skin, leaving behind the vestiges of our former lives and embracing the limitless potential of our future selves.

In these moments of transmutation, we come to understand the true nature of our existence, the undulatory and transient quality of life that implores us to seize the opportunities for personal evolution laid before us.

The art of reinvention is a testament to the indomitable spirit of humanity, the capacity for resilience and adaptation that has allowed our species to thrive amidst the upheavals of time and change. And so, let us embrace the journey of reinvention, the arduous and exhilarating process of self-discovery that illuminates the path toward personal growth and the realization of our true potential.

In the end, it is not the constancy of our being that defines us but rather our ability to adapt and develop in the face of adversity and change. It is our adeptness at reinvention, the willingness to reimagine and redefine ourselves, that serves as the bedrock upon which our personal growth and evolution are built.

⑤ The Power of Perspective

Change is an ever-present, loyal, and inescapable companion, a quirky partner with whom we must learn to collaborate if we are to navigate the complexities and mutability of our existence. It is an interaction that demands improvised coordination, the ability to shift and adapt in response to the rhythmic shapeshifts of the ever-changing landscape that surrounds us.

In this context, the power of perspective lies in its capacity to shape our understanding of and response to this inevitable relationship, to reframe our perception of change as an essential and invigorating component of life rather than a force to be feared or resisted.

By adopting such a perspective, we become active participants in a concert of transformation, harnessing the energy of change to move our lives along, infused with the rewards of growth and self-actualization.

It is said that beauty is in the beholder's eye, and so too, is the power of change. When viewed through the lens of fear and resistance, change can appear as a menacing apparition, a harbinger of chaos and destruction that threatens to upend the delicate balance of our lives. But when viewed through the prism of opportunity and growth, change becomes a catalyst for renewal and rejuvenation. This force breathes new life into our existence's stale and stagnant corners.

This shift in perspective is not a mere intellectual exercise but a visceral and deeply felt transformation that begins in the depths of our souls and radiates outward, coloring our thoughts, feelings, and actions. By learning to embrace the dance of change, we cultivate the resilience and adaptability that are the hallmarks of a well-lived life, which is not constricted by fear and resistance but freed by the winds of possibility and the promise of developmental progress.

So let us learn to harness the power of perspective and reframe our understanding of change as an essential and invigorating component of life. In this partnership, we discover the true essence of our being, the capacity for noble evolution, waiting to be awakened by the sweet and seductive song of change.

⑥ The Wisdom of Learning

As we plot our path through the many junctions and blind turns of existence, each fork in the road presents us with new challenges and opportunities. The wisdom gleaned from our experiences serves as our guide, our intuitive beacon in the darkness. The wisdom of learning is a precious gift that we gain not through the passive accumulation of facts and figures but through active and intentional engagement with the world.

If change is our most steadfast and loyal partner, a constant companion that leads us through the swirling maelstrom of experiences and emotions that form the tapestry of our existence, it is through our interactions with change that we gain the wisdom of learning, the insights, and lessons that inform and enrich our personal growth.

As we throw ourselves into the dance of change, we must learn to listen to its whispered wisdom, to attune our senses to the subtle rhythms and patterns that underlie the apparent chaos of our lives. We must learn to recognize the lessons that change brings, to distill the essence of our experiences into nuggets of wisdom that can guide and nourish our souls.

As we have seen, in this pursuit of wisdom, we must adopt a posture of humility and openness, recognizing that we are but humble students in life's vast and ever-changing classroom.

We must set aside our preconceived notions and assumptions to embrace the possibility that we may not always be correct and that there may be valuable lessons to be learned from the unlikeliest of sources.

As we navigate the twists and turns of our unique adventures, drawing upon the accumulated wisdom of our experiences to guide our steps, we become increasingly adept at moving in harmony with change. Our adaptability is enhanced, our resilience fortified, as we learn to see the world through a wider lens, to recognize the lessons and opportunities that only perspective can reveal.

So let us commit ourselves to pursue wisdom, to the cultivation of an open and humble heart that is ever ready to learn from the experiences and lessons that change brings, for it is in this spirit of inquiry and exploration that we will find the keys to unlocking the treasures of personal growth, the secrets to mastering the dance of life.

⑦ The Resilience of Acceptance

In life's vast and ever-changing theatre, we are but mere players, our roles and destinies subject to the whims and vagaries of forces beyond our control. Yet, amidst this uncertain performance, we must learn to cultivate the resilience of acceptance, surrender to the inevitability of change, and embrace its inherent unpredictability.

As we stand at the forefront of an unknown stage, gazing into the abyss of uncertainty that yawns before us, it is easy to be overwhelmed by fear and anxiety and cling to the illusion of control we so desperately crave. Yet, in these moments of doubt and trepidation, the true power of acceptance reveals itself, offering us a lifeline as the show continues onward.

To practice the art of acceptance is to relinquish our futile attempts to bend the world to our will, to surrender to the realization that there are forces and events beyond our control. It is to acknowledge that change is an intrinsic and inescapable aspect of life and that our destinies are woven from the ever-shifting threads of circumstance and fate.

This act of surrender, however, is not one of weakness or resignation but of strength and resilience. In embracing the uncertainties of life, we free ourselves from the brittleness of fear and anxiety, learning to flex and stretch as life demands.

As we cultivate the resilience of acceptance, we find ourselves better equipped to weather the storms of life, to emerge from the disruptions of change stronger and wiser than before.

The fires of adversity, our souls refined by the polish of experience, temper our hearts.

So let us practice the art of acceptance, surrendering to the inevitability of change and embracing its inherent uncertainties. Let us take to the stage with open arms and hearts, knowing that through this act of surrender, we will find the strength and wisdom to participate in the grand show of life with courage and curiosity.

⑧ The Celebration of Growth

Change is the master weaver, its nimble fingers intertwining threads of experience, emotion, and circumstance into an intricate, ever-evolving pattern. It is the force that drives our personal growth, the crucible in which our true selves are forged and refined. And it is in our recognition and celebration of this transformative power that we indeed come to understand the essential role that change plays in shaping our lives and guiding our evolution.

As we traverse the winding path of existence, we are constantly confronted with the kaleidoscopic hues of change, its shifting patterns etching indelibly upon our lives' canvas. These experiences, whether joyous or painful, triumphant or challenging, serve to mold and shape us, sculpt and delineate our character and enhance the vibrancy of our souls.

It is in these moments of transformation that we are granted the opportunity to grow, shed the layers of our former selves, and unfurl the wings of our newly emerging identity. And it is in our acknowledgment and celebration of this growth, this metamorphosis of self, that we truly come to appreciate the myriad ways in which change enriches our lives.

So join me as I raise a glass to change to the master weaver who spins the threads of our existence into a tapestry of breathtaking beauty and complexity. Let us honor the transformative power of change, acknowledging the countless ways in which it shapes our lives and guides our evolution.

As we toast, let us celebrate the personal growth that arises from our experiences with change, reveling in the triumphs and lessons that these moments of the Renaissance give us. And as we sip, let us reaffirm our commitment to embracing the ever-shifting tides of existence, to dancing with the ebb and flow of life in all its glorious and unpredictable splendor.

After all, as we glide gracefully through the emerging choreography of life, it is our ability to embrace change and adapt to its uncertainties that allows us to flourish and thrive. With the poise and elegance of a seasoned dancer, we can confidently navigate our capacity to grow, evolve, and adapt to the ever-changing rhythm of the human experience.

XXV.

Building Steadfast Resilience and Nurturing Personal Growth

As we navigate life, resilience can be seen as a gleaming armor that safeguards our inner sanctity when adversity strikes or triumph beckons. Like a steadfast warrior riding on the steed of change, the resilient individual is equipped to weather the battles and opportunities of life, emerging from each challenge with a renewed sense of purpose and a deeper understanding of their own capabilities.

❶ The Essence of Resilience

Simultaneously, resilience is the very essence that pervades our being, the indomitable force that lends us the strength and fortitude to endure the vicissitudes of existence. It is a quality as multifaceted as a diamond, its brilliant faces reflecting the innumerable ways in which we persevere in the face of adversity and rise from the ashes of defeat.

To truly appreciate the significance of resilience in shaping our lives and fostering personal growth, we must plunge deep into the depths of its complex nature, exploring the emotional, mental, and physical dimensions that coalesce to form this most essential of human attributes.

Emotional fortitude, the ability to maintain equanimity in life's turbulent seas, is a crucial facet of resilience. This inner composure enables us to withstand the gales of sorrow and the gusts of disappointment, to navigate the squalls of heartache and the storms of loss.

Mental endurance is another facet of resilience, the grit, and determination that propels us forward in the face of seemingly insurmountable challenges. The tenacity enables us to scale the imposing cliffs of our aspirations, the stubborn resolve that drives us to push through the barriers that stand between us and our goals. It is also the fuel that feeds the fire of our ambition, the relentless drive that spurs us onward in our quest for personal growth and self-actualization.

The ability to bounce back from setbacks, the capacity to rise from the depths of despair and emerge more robust and more resilient than before, is perhaps the most tangible glistening face of the diamond that is resilience.

This quality embodies the mythical phoenix, the fabled creature that rises from the flames of its own destruction, reborn and renewed. It is in our ability to rebound from adversity that the true essence of resilience is revealed, a testament to the indomitable spirit within each of us.

As you will undoubtedly have gleaned by this exhilarating point in our shared adventure toward personal growth and self-improvement, resilience is one of the many guides that can efficaciously aid our sacred journey.

By understanding the various components of resilience—emotional fortitude, mental endurance, and the ability to bounce back from setbacks—we can better appreciate its significance in shaping our lives and fostering our evolution. For it is only in adversity that the mettle of our character is tested and strengthened, the raw ore of our potential forged into the gleaming steel of our realized selves.

❷ The Crucible of Adversity

Adversity weaves its threaded additions through the very fabric of our existence, the chiaroscuro of light and shadow that defines the contours of our being. Our capacity for resilience is honed through challenge, the fires of adversity tempering our spirit and fortifying our resolve.

Like the master blacksmith who forges the unyielding steel of a finely crafted blade, adversity shapes the resilient individual, molding them into a figure of unwavering strength and indomitable determination.

As we traverse the rugged terrain of life's journey, each trial we face is an opportunity for growth and self-discovery. Though they may scorch and sear, the fires of adversity serve to anneal our spirit, hardening our resolve and focus. The relentless heat of the forge strengthens our character, burning away the impurities of doubt and fear, leaving behind a core of pure, unyielding determination.

The resilient individual, tempered by the flames of adversity, emerges from each trial with a heightened sense of self-awareness and a deepened understanding of their inner strength. Like the warrior's weapon, the resilient spirit is flexible yet unbreakable, capable of withstanding the blows of life's hammers without faltering or bending.

This paradoxical combination of pliability and steadfastness defines the essence of resilience, the equilibrium of strength and suppleness that allows us to endure and prosper.

In the confessional narrative of our lives, we often find that our most profound moments of growth arise from the remnants of our most significant challenges. The trials we face, though they may leave us battered and bruised, serve to refine our character and forge our resilience, preparing us for the battles that lie ahead.

In the crucible of adversity, we learn the accurate measure of our strength and discover the depths of our fortitude, the fires of challenge molding us into the resilient individuals we are destined to become.

Knowing this, let us see clearly the role of adversity in forging resilience, as, like tempered steel, the resilient individual is made stronger within the crucible of hardship and emerges from each trial with a heightened sense of self-awareness and certainty.

❸ The Power of Mindset

Returning to the resplendent theatre of the human experience, we find that the grand drama of our lives is unfolding with or without our active participation, a dazzling spectacle of triumphs and tragedies, of victories, won and battles lost.

However, when we step beyond the curtain and meet our struggles head-on, our character is manifested, the resilient individual emerging forth thanks to the power of mindset. This all-encompassing mental framework shapes our perceptions and guides our actions.

To cultivate a resilient mindset, one must first recognize the importance of optimism, that radiant lighthouse of hope that pierces the darkness of despair and illuminates the way for triumph's safe passage.

The resilient individual gazes upon the world through a lens of boundless possibility, seeing not the obstacles that bar their way but the opportunities that lie just beyond their grasp. It is this unshakable faith in the promise of tomorrow that sustains them through the storms of today, the unwavering belief in their ability to overcome even the most impossible odds.

In tandem with optimism, the resilient mindset is characterized by self-efficacy, the unshakable conviction in one's own abilities, and the steadfast assurance that success is within their reach.

This self-assurance is forged in the fires of experience, each trial and tribulation serving to strengthen the resilient individual's belief in their own capacity for growth and transformation. Like a master carpenter, the resilient individual hones their self-efficacy with each stroke of the hammer, birthing from their raw materials a figure of determination and resolve.

But perhaps the most vital component of the resilient mindset is an unwavering belief in one's own ability to overcome. This steadfast faith serves as the ballast that keeps the resilient individual grounded amidst the turbulence of life, the immutable certainty that they will prevail in the face of adversity. This unyielding belief allows the resilient individual to face the unexpected and emerge on the other side, battered but unbowed, their spirit stronger and more committed than ever before.

This makes cultivating a resilient mindset a worthy pursuit indeed, nurturing within ourselves the seeds of optimism, self-efficacy, and an unwavering belief in our ability to overcome obstacles.

 The Pillars of Support

Human existence allows us to take in at will the exquisite detail of a veritable panorama of passion and pain, triumph and tribulation, and, with any luck, connection, and camaraderie. In the presence of adversity, the actual potency of our support networks is revealed, a sturdy bastion within which we can rest before continuing to traverse the treacherous terrain of life's challenges.

Crucially, through the bonds of connection and camaraderie, we draw strength and inspiration during times of difficulty, our resilience nurtured and sustained by the collective power of the human spirit.

The first pillar of support, the cornerstone upon which our bastion of resilience is founded, is that of family. These unbreakable bonds of blood and kinship serve as an unyielding anchor in the storm-tossed seas of life, a safe harbor wherein we can find solace and succor from the tempests of the world. It is within the nurturing embrace of familial love that the seeds of resilience are sown, our spirits fortified by the unspoken certainties of loyalty and devotion that define the ties that bind.

Next, the pillar of friendship, a loyal friend, is a salve for the soul, a brightness shining through the darkness of despair, and a steadfast ally in the face of adversity.

Through the shared experiences of joy and sorrow, laughter and tears, the bonds of friendship are forged and strengthened, the resilient individual reinvigorated by the unwavering support of their trusted confidants.

And then there is the pillar of the community, that interconnected web of relationships that spans the vast expanse of our social landscape. Within the community network, we find a plethora of diverse perspectives and experiences that can inform and enrich our understanding of the world, the resilient individual drawing upon this vast reservoir of collective wisdom in their quest for personal growth.

By immersing ourselves in the nurturing embrace of community, we create a foundation upon which our resilience can thrive, the bonds of connection and camaraderie serving as a bulwark against uncertainty.

Last, the pillar of mentorship, the tradition of guidance and sage counsel, is passed down from generation to generation. Through the tutelage of our mentors, we collect invaluable insights and lessons, their hard-won wisdom serving as a guiding light on our path to resilience.

So, let us acknowledge the importance of a strong support network in nurturing resilience and endeavor to surround ourselves with a community of individuals who uplift and encourage us.

Through the bonds of connection and camaraderie, we draw strength and inspiration during times of difficulty, our resilience flourishing amidst the fertile soil of love, loyalty, and shared experience.

5. The Art of Adaptation

Existence, a ceaseless waltz between the ephemeral and the eternal, calls upon us in perpetuity to adapt and transform our lives, an ever-evolving and increasingly complex tapestry of change and growth. The art of adaptation, then, is a skill that must be refined, a skilled craft that requires the utmost finesse and talent as we learn to navigate the capricious currents of life's vast and turbulent ocean.

Picture, if you will, a master mariner, the seasoned captain of a stately ship that traverses the high seas. His gaze fixed resolutely upon the horizon as he adjusts his sails in response to the shifting winds.

This skilled seafarer, a paragon of adaptability, understands the fickle nature of the elements and embraces the inherent uncertainty that accompanies each journey. He knows that, in order to stay afloat amidst the tossing and turning waters of existence, he must cultivate the resilience needed to adapt and persevere.

The first step in honing the art of adaptation is to recognize and accept the inevitability of change. Like the seasons that wax and wane, change is a fundamental aspect of the human experience, an omnipresent force that defines the very essence of our existence. When we embrace change as an opportunity for growth and transformation, instead of fearing or resisting it, we cultivate the resilience needed to stay afloat amidst life's turbulent waters.

Next, we must learn to adjust our sails in the face of shifting winds, developing the flexibility and open-mindedness necessary to adapt to new circumstances and challenges. This mental suppleness, akin to the graceful bend of a tree's limb in the face of a gale, allows us to withstand the relentless onslaught of life's disruptions, our spirits remaining afloat thanks to the resilience that arises from our ability to adapt and persevere.

And finally, we must seek wisdom and guidance from the experiences and lessons that change brings, using these insights to inform and enrich our personal growth. As we navigate the unpredictable currents of life's vast ocean, we can draw upon this accumulated wisdom to guide our course, our resilience strengthened by the knowledge that we have weathered the storms of the past and emerged stronger and wiser for the experience.

Thus, let us hone the art of adaptation, learning to embrace change and uncertainty as opportunities for growth and transformation. By developing the ability to adjust our sails in the face of shifting winds, we cultivate the resilience needed to stay afloat amidst life's expansive waters.

❻ The Practice of Self-Compassion

It is safe to say that, in life, we are often our own harshest critics, subjecting ourselves to an unrelenting barrage of self-censure and reproach. Yet, amidst the cacophony of self-flagellation, we must embrace self-compassion, treating ourselves with kindness and understanding during times of struggle as we journey along the winding path of personal growth and self-discovery.

For a moment, imagine a tender sapling buffeted by the elements, its fragile branches quivering in the face of raging circumstances. To nurture and protect this fledgling tree, we must provide the sustenance and support it requires to grow and flourish, cultivating a sanctuary of warmth, love, and understanding in which it may thrive.

Similarly, we must cultivate a wellspring of self-compassion, a refuge from self-doubt and criticism that may otherwise threaten to lay waste to our sense of self-worth and self-acceptance.

The practice of self-compassion begins with recognizing our own intrinsic value and acknowledging our shared humanity. First, we must understand that, like the many other souls who traverse the earth, we are all fallible beings, susceptible to the vagaries of existence and the occasional misstep on the path to self-improvement.

By extending to ourselves the same kindness and understanding that we would offer to a beloved friend or family member, we create a sanctuary of self-compassion within which our resilience may grow and flourish.

Moreover, we must learn to relinquish the paralyzing grip of perfectionism, accepting the inherent imperfections that define the human experience. In this act of radical self-acceptance, we free ourselves from self-criticism and self-doubt, allowing our spirits to soar on the wings of self-compassion, elevated by the knowledge that we are enough, just as we are.

And finally, we must seek solace in the knowledge that, through the practice of self-compassion, we are cultivating an abundant reserve of resilience that enables us to persevere through life's challenges.

As we nurture this sense of self-worth and self-acceptance, we create the foundation upon which our resilience can thrive, empowering us to align within ourselves a deep-rooted belief in our own inherent worth. To claim such a mighty prize, enacting self-compassion begins simply with enacting self-awareness and choosing to treat ourselves with kindness and understanding during times of struggle.

❼ The Quest for Personal Growth

On the next leg of our noble quest for personal growth and self-improvement, we are presented with a sequence of opportunities for learning and self-discovery. Unfortunately, amidst the hither and thither of adventure, it is all too easy to lose sight of our true purpose, becoming entangled in the web of distraction and disillusionment.

Yet, it is precisely in these moments of uncertainty that we must remain steadfast in our pursuit, our gaze fixed firmly upon the horizon of self-actualization as we navigate the ever-changing landscape of life.

To maintain this unwavering commitment to our own evolution, we must first acknowledge that the path to personal growth is neither linear nor predictable. Rather, it is a meandering journey, fraught with obstacles and setbacks, triumphs and tribulations, a rich medley of experiences that serve to shape and refine our character, like water flowing across the smooth surface of an ancient stone.

Faced with adversity, we must view each challenge as an opportunity for growth. Like the intrepid explorer who braves the uncharted wilderness, we must embrace the unknown, undeterred by the possibility of failure and encouraged by the knowledge that it is through these trials that we emerge stronger, wiser, and more resilient.

Furthermore, we must cultivate a mindset of curiosity and open-mindedness, approaching each new experience with the wide-eyed wonder of a child, eager to learn and unencumbered by the constraints of preconceived notions.

In this spirit of inquiry, we are afforded the opportunity to examine our beliefs and assumptions, to challenge the paradigms that govern our lives, and to embark upon a journey of self-discovery that illuminates the hidden recesses of our souls.

As we forge ahead on this quest for personal growth, let us also remember, once more, to celebrate our progress, to honor the milestones we achieve and the lessons we glean from our experiences. In this way, we reaffirm our commitment to our evolution, providing the sustenance and nourishment necessary to sustain our spirits and fuel our continued growth.

⑧ The Celebration of Resilience

As we look back upon the intricate motifs of personal growth that we have woven into the tapestries of our lives thus far, one cannot overlook the significance of resilience, that ineffable quality that has steered us loyally in creating a pattern that embodies self-discovery. As we continue in our composition, it is only fitting to pause to celebrate and honor the resilience that has served us well, guiding us at blind turns and unsignposted junctions.

To truly appreciate the magnitude of this celebration, we must first unpack the notion of resilience, exploring its multidimensional nature and the myriad of ways in which it has shaped our lives.

Like the finest coffee blend, resilience is composed of a harmonious balance. Still, rather than being of the fruits of rugged mountains and rich valleys, this blend is one of emotional fortitude, mental endurance, and the capacity to rebound from setbacks, each note resonating in perfect harmony with the others, creating an irresistible and heady aroma of strength and determination.

In honoring the resilience we have cultivated throughout our journey, we must also acknowledge adversity's role. Through the heat and pressure of challenge, resilience's flavors meet maturity, emerging stronger and more durable, imbued with the wisdom and self-awareness that can only be gained when conditions force transformation.

As we celebrate our resilience, let us also recognize the ways in which it has propelled us toward personal growth, serving as both anchor and sail in our voyage through the vast and unpredictable seas of existence.

Faced with uncertainty, our resilience grants us the courage to confront our fears and the tenacity to surmount the obstacles that stand in our path, imbuing us with the confidence and self-assurance necessary to chart our course toward self-actualization.

Moreover, this celebration serves to reaffirm the importance of resilience in guiding our journey, a timely reminder of the indomitable spirit that dwells within each of us, waiting to be summoned in times of need.

By recognizing the value of resilience, we honor our progress and rekindle the flames of determination and hope that burn within our souls, fueling our continued pursuit of personal growth and self-discovery.

> **In conclusion, let us take the time to honor resilience, that formidable force that has guided us so astutely. By celebrating the resilience we have cultivated throughout our journey, we acknowledge how it has shaped our lives and propelled us toward personal growth, reaffirming its importance in steering our voyage through the vast and unpredictable seas of existence.**

XXVI.

Practical Strategies for Reigniting Inner Evolution

In the composition of our daily lives, the many aspects we have explored thus far mount a harmonious melody that imbues a profound sense of meaning and purpose.

As we become composers of greater accomplishment, we must seize the power to transmute the base metals of adversity into the golden essence of yet more of the qualities we wish to grow, reinforcing our inner strength and cultivating our capacity for self-improvement. In this chapter, we shall accustom ourselves to practical strategies to guide us through constant reinvigoration.

① Cultivating Greater Self-Awareness:

As we embark upon the rigorous yet exhilarating journey of self-discovery, we must pause periodically to cultivate the soils of our self-awareness, tilling and turning in introspection, curiosity, and compassion.

These soils must never be allowed to turn barren because it is within this hallowed ground that we nurture a profound understanding of our thoughts, emotions, and beliefs, each delicate sprout of knowledge unfurling to reveal the intricate nature of our true potential.

To foster such a deep and abiding sense of self-awareness, we must approach our inner garden with the gentle touch of a master horticulturist that is ever in step with the seasons, tending to the tendrils of our thoughts and the blossoms of our emotions with the same tender care and attention that we would afford to the most fragile and exquisite flowering tree, that casts its petals further with each passing year.

By examining the inner workings of our minds with a curious and compassionate eye, we may also begin to identify the random but sacred patterns and motifs that define our existence, bringing them to light and allowing them to inform our personal growth and resilience.

In this quiet introspection, we may extend the groundwork for resilience by identifying growth areas and pruning away the deadwood of outdated beliefs and fallacies hindering our progress. Like a skilled gardener who expertly shapes the branches of a bonsai tree, we must learn to recognize and nurture the buds of potential that lie dormant within our souls, coaxing them forth with the gentle warmth of self-compassion and the nourishing light of self-acceptance.

As we continue to cultivate self-awareness, we also create ideal conditions for the germination of resilience, allowing it to take root and flourish amidst the verdant foliage of our expanding inner landscape. Through introspection, we foster the growth of resilience by recognizing and understanding our unique strengths and weaknesses and the multitude of ways in which our thoughts and emotions shape our lives.

In conclusion, cultivating self-awareness builds the soil that nourishes our quest for resilience and personal growth. By fostering a deep understanding of our inner world and tending to the garden of our thoughts, emotions, and beliefs with curiosity and compassion, we lay the groundwork for resilience and unlock the boundless potential that dwells within each of us.

In this oasis of self-awareness, we may nurture boundless personal growth, unfurling and blossoming into the resplendent manifestation of our potential.

② Meeting Change With Confidence

As change becomes a veteran compatriot, we see the transient and ever-changing nature of existence with greater clarity, allowing the fluidity of change to wash over us like the soothing caress of a gentle tide. In the eye of change, we discover our innate capacity for resilience and adaptability. These same qualities enable us to navigate the capricious currents of fortune and fate with grace and aplomb.

To further develop our flexible mindset, we must relinquish our futile attempts to grasp at the billowing nebulosity of certainty, in full recognition that change is not a cruel interloper to be feared or resisted but rather an integral and natural component of the human experience.

With each passing moment, the shapeshifting silhouette of existence spins and transmutes, the vibrant sensory elements of our lives blending and morphing in a ceaseless dance of transformation.

By welcoming the impermanent nature of life, we cultivate the adaptability necessary for building resilience and traversing the unfamiliar landscape of existence.

As we immerse ourselves fully, we may begin to see the beauty in the fleeting nature of existence, the delicate interplay of light and shadow that defines the human experience. It is within this embrace of change that we find the fertile ground for personal growth and self-discovery, our hearts and minds expanding to encompass the boundless potential that lies hidden within each transformative moment.

③ Reaffirming Realistic Goals

When striving for personal growth, it is paramount to set realistic and achievable goals, for these quantified ambitions illuminate our way forward with the steadfast glow of purpose and direction.

With that in mind, there is always time to revisit the goals that serve as the milestones of our progress on this journey, the tangible manifestations of our deepest desires and aspirations, beckoning us ever onward as we strive to achieve our fullest potential.

Now far better equipped to mount a successful process of introspection, we can delve yet more profound into the hidden recesses of our souls to uncover our most cherished values and aspirations. It is upon this ever-expanding foundation of self-knowledge that we can continue to round and shape our goals, ensuring that they align with our most authentic selves and embody the essence of our dreams.

In crafting our goals, we must strike a delicate balance between ambition and realism, allowing our aspirations to soar while remaining firmly grounded in the realm of the attainable. To this end, we must distill our long-term objectives into manageable tasks, a series of incremental steps that, when taken in succession, bring us ever closer to the realization of our dreams.

By re-evaluating and honing realistic expectations, freshly emboldened by our awaking resilience, we foster a sense of purpose and maintain momentum on our journey toward personal growth. This, in turn, nurtures the adaptability and fortitude required to overcome obstacles and embrace the transformative power of change.

In essence, setting realistic goals is akin to charting a course that leads us, step by step, toward the fulfillment of our deepest desires and aspirations. By harnessing wisdom and resilience to hone achievable objectives that align with our values and dreams, we imbue our journey with renewed purpose and direction, cultivating the resilience and adaptability needed to weather the storms of life and emerge stronger, wiser, and more self-aware.

④ Nurturing a Growth Mindset

There is more that we can do to cultivate a growth mindset. With each shift in perspective, we can further reframe our understanding of life's obstacles and setbacks.

Rather than perceiving these challenges as vast mountains, we will increasingly begin to see them as modest stepping stones, each one offering a unique opportunity for personal evolution and self-discovery. By embracing the growth process, we empower ourselves to persevere through adversity, bolstered by the knowledge that each trial serves to strengthen our character and enhance our capacity for resilience.

As we journey along the path of personal development, we must remain vigilant in our quest for growth, actively seeking out opportunities to enhance our perspective and expanding our knowledge, skills, and self-awareness. To develop a growth mindset, we must remain open to feedback and actively embrace constructive criticism. We should recognize that challenges test our true mettle and forge our potential for greatness.

When we view life's inevitable difficulties through the lens of a growth mindset, we transform them into gateways for growth. Each challenge invites us to pave the way for a more authentic, self-aware, and fulfilling existence.

⑤ Strengthening a Vibrant Support Network

When cultivating a community of kindred spirits, it is vital to seek out those individuals whose values and aspirations resonate with our own, knowing that these parallels may subtly shift and evolve over time but that a strong support network's resilience lies in structural integrity rather than any singular presence.

Those within such a sphere offer a sense of solace and understanding as we traverse the arduous path of personal growth. In the company of these like-minded souls, we are afforded the opportunity to share our triumphs and tribulations, our joys and sorrows, forging bonds of mutual support that serve as a bulwark against life's storms.

As we further build and widen our support network, it is essential that we nurture these relationships with care and intention, for it is through the act of reciprocity that the roots of camaraderie grow deep and strong. Moreover, by offering our support and encouragement to those within our circle, we foster an environment of trust and vulnerability, a safe harbor in which we may lay bare our doubts and fears, secure in the knowledge that we are not alone in our struggles.

In moments of darkness and despair, when the weight of adversity threatens to break our resolve, the support network emerges as a raft, elegantly riding the turbulent waters of life with a steady and unwavering spirit. Thus, as we continue to dance upon the stage of life, let us remember that we must cultivate a strong support network just as we tend to our inner resilience. A circle of trusted confidants can offer encouragement, guidance, and camaraderie during times of difficulty.

⑥ Practicing Mindfulness and Self-Compassion

In life, where the drama of existence unfolds in a whirlwind of emotion and experience, we may still find ourselves swept up in the tumultuous currents of our thoughts and feelings despite an intention of mindfulness. Yet, amidst this chaos, a re-grounding remains dependent on the arts of mindfulness and self-compassion.

To re-engage in regular mindfulness practice, we must first re-attune ourselves to a non-judgmental awareness of the present moment, observing the comings and goings of our thoughts and emotions with the detachment of a disinterested spectator.

In this state of unadulterated presence, we bear witness to how our inner world is meeting external stimuli, releasing any unwelcome fleeting expression of our transient nature so that we may become calm again.

As we hone our ability to dwell in the present, we are reminded of the transformative power of self-compassion, a gentle balm that soothes the wounds of our fragile psyche.

By treating ourselves with kindness and understanding during these times of struggle, we create a nurturing environment where our resilience may reemerge and thrive.

In our most vulnerable moments, when the weight of self-doubt and insecurity threatens to shatter our resolve, it is the practice of mindfulness and self-compassion that emerges as our steadfast ally. By attending to the delicate whispers of our heart, we learn to embrace the full spectrum of our human experience, our tender self-compassion gently reminding us that we can endure far more than we would once have imagined.

⑦ Fostering Further Gratitude and Positivity

Within life's experiences, where threads of joy and sorrow weave an intricate pattern, the radiant hues of gratitude and positivity bring color and vitality to our existence. As we traverse the human condition's labyrinthine paths, the deliberate cultivation of these qualities illuminates the way forward, casting an unmistakable radiance upon the road less traveled.

To foster a mighty attitude of gratitude, one must repeat the practice of pausing to take stock of the myriad blessings that adorn our lives, each a precious jewel that gleams with the light of a thousand suns. From the simple pleasures of a fragrant cup of tea to the profound connections we share with our loved ones, we unearth a deep and abiding sense of contentment and satisfaction in recognizing these gifts.

As we nurture this sense of gratitude, we soon find that a burgeoning positivity, a radiant optimism that infuses our every endeavor with renewed enthusiasm and vigor, accompanies it. By focusing our attention on the aspects of life that bring us joy and fulfillment, we create a fertile ground in which the seeds of happiness may take root and flourish.

When the storm clouds of adversity gather on the horizon, it is the resilient spirit of gratitude and positivity that shelters us from the tempestuous onslaught. By actively maintaining an optimistic outlook, we summon forth the emotional resilience necessary to overcome life's challenges and setbacks and ensure that our comfort will be greater when future storms arise.

So, let us embrace the practice of gratitude and positivity with enthusiasm and conviction, for it is in the continued cultivation of these radiant qualities that we discover the bottomless nature of our resilience. As we voyage onward, the brilliance of gratitude and positivity guides us toward realizing our most cherished dreams and aspirations.

⑧ Prioritizing Self-Care and Well-Being

We often find ourselves playing myriad parallel roles in this life, each demanding our unyielding commitment and tireless devotion. Amidst this miscellany of responsibility and duty, it is all too easy to lose sight of the importance of self-care and well-being, the stable core around which our resilience and fortitude rotate.

To truly master the art of self-nurturing, we must remind ourselves frequently of the indispensability of our own well-being, for it is the act of prioritizing our physical, emotional, and mental health that ensures the longevity of our resilience. This essential ingredient sustains us through the ebb and flow of life's tides.

In the quest for self-care, we must seek out activities that nourish our souls and rejuvenate our spirits, indulging in the soothing balm of relaxation and the refreshing tonic of self-expression. Whether it be the gentle caress of a yoga mat, the lilting melodies of a beloved instrument, or the fragrant embrace of a resplendent garden, it is in these pursuits that we find solace and sanctuary from the relentless demands of the world.

As we dedicate time and energy to our well-being, we soon discover that it is not a luxury, but a necessity, for it is in the cultivation of our inner sanctum that we lay the groundwork for resilience. Self-care fortifies our emotional ramparts and strengthens our mental resolve, ensuring that we are well-equipped to weather the storms that inevitably arise.

So let us make a solemn pledge to double down upon our prioritization of self-care and well-being, nurturing the garden of our souls with the tender ministrations of love and compassion. Only through this act of tending to our own needs can we establish a foundation upon which our resilience can thrive, a mighty fortress from which we may face the trials and tribulations of life with courage and conviction.

⑨ Reflecting on Progress and Growth

In life, where our triumphs and tribulations intertwine to form the intricate narrative of our existence, it is vital that we take stock of the progress we have made in the relentless pursuit of self-improvement with dogged regularity. The act of reflection, like a silvered mirror held to our souls, allows us to glimpse the depths of our being, revealing both the victories and the setbacks that have shaped our journey.

To make a habit of meaningful introspection, we must cultivate the patience and humility necessary to confront the truth of our past and our past truths. In this process, we cast a discerning eye over our lives, acknowledging the peaks and valleys delineating our path. Finally, we celebrate our achievements with exultant pride, honoring our determination and resilience, propelling us toward greatness.

Yet, in equal measure, we must also contend with our setbacks, those moments where we faltered and stumbled, our dreams shrouded by doubt. It is in these lowlands of shadow that we find our most profound lessons;

the wisdom gleaned from repeated confrontation with adversity. Through this process of self-examination, we emerge with a deeper understanding of our strengths and vulnerabilities, as well as a renewed commitment to our evolution.

> **Of course, we also gain clarity on our present trajectory, honing our sense of purpose and direction in pursuing resilience and personal growth. This clarity creates a living chronicle of our journey, a testament to our unwavering commitment to resilience and self-improvement.**

XXVII.

The Eternal Learning of the Mirrored Soul

Like the intricate gilt frame of a finely crafted mirror, the human soul possesses a complex depth that reflects the richness of our inner lives. However, to embark upon the path of personal growth, one must channel the flawless finish of the mirror itself instead, engaging in quiet self-reflection, learning from experiences, and seeking support from others.

In this chapter, we shall reflect upon the significance of these essential practices, examining how they guide us toward a deeper understanding of ourselves and a more profound connection with the world.

① The Power of Self-Reflection

Within every individual's inner world lies a boundless expanse, a realm of profound self-discovery that invites the brave to explore its depths. In repeating this introspective odyssey, we truly master the art of self-reflection. This practice serves as both a compass and a remedy for the soul, guiding us higher into the mountains of personal growth and self-actualization.

As we turn our gaze inward, examining the complex tapestry of thoughts, emotions, and motivations that comprise our beings we inevitably find new and unexpected shadowy corners of our consciousness, uncovering our strengths and weaknesses, triumphs, and follies.

We confront our fears and vulnerabilities, acknowledging the scars and blemishes that serve as poignant reminders of our human frailty. Yet, in equal measure, we celebrate the sheer scale and scope of our explorations, those that have allowed us to gain the tools necessary to chart a course toward a more fulfilling and authentic existence.

By committing to a practice of frequent self-reflection, we embark on a lifelong journey of introspection and self-discovery, navigating the ever-shifting seas of our inner world with steadfast resolve.

Through this sacred communion with the self, we come to know ourselves more intimately, forging an unbreakable bond with the essence of our being and the boundless potential that lies within.

And so, I encourage you to take up the mantle of the self-reflective explorer, venturing into the uncharted realms of our consciousness with a courageous heart and an open mind. Through this fearless quest, we unlock the secrets of our souls, gaining insight into our thoughts, emotions, and motivations, allowing us to understand better our strengths, weaknesses, and areas of potential growth.

2. Learning from Experiences

In the vast intricacies of existence, each moment, each encounter, and each breath we take adds another delicate strand to the elaborate masterpiece that is our lives. Yet, within these intricacies, we uncover the hidden lessons that shape our character, guide our journey, and ultimately mold us into the individuals we are destined to become.

As we meander onward, each time triumphs or tribulations beset us, we will be ready to draw upon the chiaroscuro of our prior experiences, painting in our informed response a vivid tableau that reflects the complexities of our human nature.

In the melting pot of experience, we forge our resilience and wisdom, emerging from life's challenges as more refined and enlightened versions of ourselves.

With each step we take, we are given a choice: to embrace the full spectrum of our experiences or to shy away from the darkness that often accompanies the light.

In choosing the former, we unlock the boundless potential that lies within the heart of every human being. Through the embrace of our experiences, both the radiant and the shadowed, we come to understand the true nature of our existence.

As we delve into the recesses of our memories, we uncover the pearls of wisdom that yearn to be discovered. We learn from our failures as much as from our successes. Each misstep is a gentle reminder of the fragility and beauty of the human condition. In acknowledging and building upon these lessons, we cultivate a spirit of humility and a thirst for self-improvement, fulfillment, authenticity, and enlightened grace.

❸ Finding Sanctuary in the Support of Others

As we have explored, great power exists in the intricate web of relationships that bind us together. Innately social creatures, we are drawn to the warmth and comfort of human connection, which creates an invisible thread that links us across time and space.

Within the interlacing networks of these connections lies a treasure trove of wisdom, a wealth of knowledge and experience that transcends the boundaries of our individual lives, a gentle reminder that we are not alone in our journey towards self-discovery and personal growth.

We often find ourselves yearning for the companionship and guidance of those who share our path. In continuously seeking the support of others who align with our aspirations, we open ourselves to a symphony of ideas, perspectives, and experiences that enrich our understanding.

The conversations that unfold, the laughter that bubbles forth, and the tears that are shed all contribute to the intricate mosaic of our existence, fostering a sense of empathy and connection that strengthens our resilience and fuels our personal growth.

The gentle touch of a friend's hand upon our shoulder, the whispered words of encouragement from a loved one, or the knowing glance shared between two souls all serve to remind us of the power of human connection.

In these moments of intimacy, we glimpse the essence of our shared humanity, the common threads that bind us together in a tapestry of love, compassion, and understanding. Through these connections, we come to recognize the universal nature of our struggles, the shared aspirations that guide our journey, and the collective wisdom that illuminates our path.

To seek support from others is to acknowledge our vulnerability and embrace the fragility and beauty of our human condition. In reaching out to those around us, we learn to accept the outstretched hands of others, allowing the ebb and flow of love and support to wash over us, nourishing our souls and nurturing our resilience.

It is through the warmth of constantly nurtured human connection that we come to understand the true nature of our existence. This existence is at once unique and universal, a delicate balance of light and shadow, joy and sorrow.

So let us weave that communal web into our tapestries, embracing the exchange of ideas, perspectives, and experiences that enrich our understanding, for it is in the company of our fellow travelers that we find the strength and resilience to navigate the winding path toward personal growth, a journey that is both solitary and shared.

④ The Symbiosis of Self-Reflection and External Support

I bid you make a formal introduction between your two allies, self-reflection, and external support because these natural dance partners are destined to move in harmony, their steps an exquisite choreography that guides us towards a deeper understanding of ourselves and our place within the world.

The art of self-reflection, a contemplative act of introspection, invites us to tour the recesses of our minds, exploring the caverns of our thoughts, emotions, and beliefs with a curious and compassionate eye. Through this process, we uncover the gems of self-awareness, the shimmering truths hidden beneath the surface, waiting to be discovered and cherished.

Yet, as we waltz through the halls of introspection, we must not forget the importance of our fellow dancers, those trusted companions who accompany us on our journey toward enlightenment.

In seeking the guidance and support of others, we open ourselves to a wealth of wisdom and experience that transcends the confines of our individual lives. Moreover, exchanging ideas, perspectives, and experiences enriches our understanding, offering us a window into the minds and hearts of those who share our path.

The symbiosis of self-reflection and external support creates a dynamic interplay, a concordant balance that fosters both self-awareness and communal connection. In this fine pairing, we find the transformative power of introspection and human connection united, a synergy that facilitates authenticity that transcends the inner landscape.

So embrace the duality of the power of self-reflection and the warmth of human connection, the twin forces that forge our resilience and propel us toward a more fulfilling and meaningful existence. By engaging in self-reflection and seeking the guidance of others, we create a dynamism that is far greater than either might forge on their own.

⑤ The Ever-Evolving Journey of Personal Growth

As we navigate the vast and unpredictable seas of personal growth with increasingly admirable skill, our journey rewards us with constant discovery and transformation. In the style of a grand symphony, our lives unfold in a series of movements, each one a reflection of our ever-evolving understanding of ourselves and the life we have learned to conquer.

The process of self-reflection, akin to the gentle caress of a maestro's baton, directs the music of our lives, inviting us to delve deep within the chambers of our hearts and minds. With each introspective note, we unearth the buried treasures of our experiences, beliefs, and emotions, allowing the melody of self-awareness to resonate through our very core.

Yet, as we traverse the symphonic landscape of self-discovery, we must not forget the harmonious contributions of our fellow musicians, those trusted companions who offer their guidance, support, and camaraderie in our times of need.

Through the exchange of ideas, perspectives, and experiences, we create a glorious orchestra of human connection. This magnificent symphony reverberates throughout our lives and enriches our understanding of the world.

The ever-evolving journey of personal growth is a perpetual composition, a layered soundscape of introspection and engagement with the world around us. As we progress through the movements of our lives, we continually refine our steps, embracing the dynamic interplay between self-reflection, learning from experiences, and seeking support from others.

> **By surrendering ourselves to this constant process of growth and transformation, we open ourselves to the boundless potential for personal evolution, charting a course toward a richer, more fulfilling existence. So let us appreciate the soaring crescendo of self-discovery and personal growth that carries us to new heights of enlightenment and authenticity.**

Epilogue

The Dawning Horizon of Self-Discovery

As we stand atop the highest peak that our perception allows thus far, the generous curve of the horizon marks the culmination of our odyssey through mindfulness, acceptance, and personal growth. In this epilogue, we shall gaze back upon the winding path we have traversed to reach such heights and contemplate the myriad lessons gleaned along the way.

Throughout this volume, we have journeyed together through the hallowed halls of introspection, gleaning invaluable insights into the complexities of the human spirit. Next, we have explored the transformative power of mindfulness, unraveling the intricacies of the present moment and discovering its profound impact on our lives. Finally, we have delved into the depths of acceptance, learning to reconcile with our past and embrace future uncertainties.

We have discovered the transformative power of the present moment, a beacon of light that illuminates our path and dispels the shadows of doubt and uncertainty. We have learned that the eternal now serves as an anchor, grounding us amidst the turbulent seas of life, and as a compass, guiding our steps toward a more fulfilling and meaningful existence.

In the words of the venerable philosopher Seneca, "The entire future lies in uncertainty: live immediately." As we strive to heed this sage counsel, let us not forget the importance of remaining ever-mindful of the present moment, for it is within the confines of the here and now that we may uncover the wellspring of wisdom, strength, and potential that lives within each of us.

Emboldened and enlivened by such thoughts and adventures, we have also traversed the landscape of personal growth, seeking to cultivate empathy, compassion, and resilience as we navigate the ever-changing tapestry of life. With each step along this path, we have encountered moments of revelation, uncovering hidden aspects of our being and opening ourselves to the boundless potential for self-discovery and transformation.

And now, as we stand at the threshold of a new dawn, we find ourselves poised to embark upon an even greater journey—a journey that transcends the confines of the written word and propels us into the realm of lived experience.

The truest essence of this odyssey lies not in the ink and parchment that document our passage but in the immeasurable wisdom that we carry forth into the world as we set sail upon the sea of life.

In the spirit of camaraderie and shared exploration, I extend an open invitation to you, dear reader, to continue nurturing your personal growth and self-improvement. May the lessons of mindfulness, acceptance, and resilience serve as steadfast companions, guiding your steps as you forge a more fulfilling and meaningful life amidst the ever-shifting tapestry of existence.

As you close this volume and set forth on your journey in self-discovery, remember that the path to personal growth and self-improvement is not solitary.

Indeed, it is a path we tread together as fellow travelers on the road to enlightenment. Therefore, I encourage you to share the insights and wisdom gleaned from these pages with those who walk beside you so that they, too, might partake in the transformative power of the present moment and find solace in the garden of self-actualization.

And so, let us bid adieu to the pages of this tome by drawing from the wisdom of the great poet John Keats: "A thing of beauty is a joy forever."

It is my hope that the beauty of our shared voyage through mindfulness, acceptance, and personal growth will continue to thread ever more resplendent detail into your unique tapestry, serving as a source of enduring joy and illuminating the path toward a more prosperous, more fulfilling existence.

Our Vision

In the present digital age, an era characterized by immediate access to a boundless array of information, we find ourselves in an ocean of opinions. While this wealth of data may satiate our curiosity on a superficial level, it often fails to provide the depth of understanding we crave—the kind of fundamental understanding that gives birth to a conscientious and comprehensive perception of the world. This is precisely where Mekiki Magazine comes into play. We stand as a beacon in the information storm, offering not just information but knowledge, wisdom, and insight.

At Mekiki Magazine, we believe in intertwining cutting-edge technology with the wisdom of industry experts to curate highly tailored content. With the integration of our unique proprietary content, we are revolutionizing how knowledge is disseminated, making it much more accessible globally. Our innovative approach harnesses technology to deliver insights that cater to global preferences and needs. We are committed to empowering our writers with advanced intelligence capabilities, both generative and predictive, to enhance their understanding of the interests of our readers.

This, in turn, allows them to deliver content that truly resonates with their audience, providing unparalleled depth and value.

At Mekiki Magazine, we are not just about informing; we are about transforming understanding, one reader at a time.

Our mission is to break down the walls between specialists and the broader audience, making all topics accessible and engaging to all. Each of our publications, whether a magazine, book, or online article, acts as a unique portal into realms of knowledge. We are not simply content creators but translators of intricate subjects, transforming abstract ideas into comprehensible, engaging narratives. In essence, we aim to fill the gap between information and understanding. At Mekiki Magazine, our readers do not just learn—they comprehend. They do not just read—they engage. And in doing so, they gain a richer, more nuanced view of the world around them.

Join us on a transformative journey of discovery with Mekiki Magazine, where cutting-edge technology merges with timeless wisdom to illuminate new horizons of knowledge and understanding.

Our Vision

Unraveling the Self: A Path to Personal Growth

Author's Bibliography

Astrid Auxier is a writer with a diverse range of published works. Through her thought-provoking work, she has resonated with readers across continents seeking inspiration and transformation. Below is a selection of Astrid Auxier's notable books:

"Unraveling the Self: A Path to Personal Growth" (2023)

A guidebook for personal growth and achieving a harmonious balance in life.

"Imperfection Illuminated: Unveiling Japanese Wisdom for a Balanced Life" (2023)

A transformative exploration of the ancient Japanese philosophies of Ikigai, Wabi-Sabi, and Kaizen.

For a complete list of Astrid Auxier's published works, please visit her official website: www.astridauxier.com

For inquiries, speaking engagements, or media requests, please contact Astrid Auxier via email at info@astridauxier.com